FEMALE DOCTORS IN CANADA

Experience and Culture

Edited by Earle Waugh, Shelley Ross, and Shirley Schipper

Female Doctors in Canada is an accessible collection of articles by experienced physicians and researchers exploring how systems, practices, and individuals might change as the ratio of practising physicians shifts from predominantly male to predominantly female. How will issues such as work hours, caregiving, and doctor-patient relationships be affected?

Canadian medical education and health care systems have been based on structures designed by and for men, influencing how women practise, what type of medicine they choose to practise, and how they wish to balance their personal lives with their work. With the goal of opening up a larger conversation, *Female Doctors in Canada* reconsiders medical education, health systems, and expectations in light of the changing face of medicine.

Highlighting the particular experience of women working in the medical profession, the editors trace the history of female practitioners in Canada, while also providing a perspective on the contemporary struggles female doctors face as they navigate a system that was originally tailored to the male experience and that has yet to be modified.

EARLE WAUGH is Director Emeritus of the Centre for Health and Culture in the Department of Family Medicine at the University of Alberta.

SHELLEY ROSS is an associate professor in the Department of Family Medicine at the University of Alberta.

SHIRLEY SCHIPPER is an associate professor in the Department of Family Medicine at the University of Alberta.

Female Doctors in Canada

Experience and Culture

EDITED BY EARLE WAUGH, SHELLEY ROSS, AND SHIRLEY SCHIPPER

UNIVERSITY OF TORONTO PRESS
Toronto Buffalo London

Toronto Buffalo London
utorontopress.com
Printed in Canada

ISBN 978-1-4875-0425-0 (cloth) ISBN 978-1-4875-2322-0 (paper)

Printed on acid-free, 100% post-consumer recycled paper with vegetable-based inks.

Library and Archives Canada Cataloguing in Publication

Female doctors in Canada : experience and culture / edited by Earle Waugh, Shelley Ross, and Shirley Schipper.

Includes bibliographical references and index.
ISBN 978-1-4875-0425-0 (cloth). ISBN 978-1-4875-2322-0 (paper)

1. Women in medicine – Canada. 2. Women physicians – Canada. 3. Medical education – Sex differences – Canada. 4. Women medical students – Canada. 5. Professional socialization – Sex differences – Canada. I. Waugh, Earle H., 1936–, editor II. Ross, Shelley, 1970–, editor III. Schipper, Shirley, editor

R692.F43 2019 610.82 C2018-905259-7

University of Toronto Press acknowledges the financial assistance to its publishing program of the Canada Council for the Arts and the Ontario Arts Council, an agency of the Government of Ontario.

Canada Council for the Arts Conseil des Arts du Canada

ONTARIO ARTS COUNCIL
CONSEIL DES ARTS DE L'ONTARIO
an Ontario government agency
un organisme du gouvernement de l'Ontario

Funded by the Government of Canada Financé par le gouvernement du Canada

Canada

FSC www.fsc.org MIX Paper from responsible sources FSC® C016245

To all the pioneer women in medicine, as well as all the women currently practising and training in medicine.

Contents

Preface: Why a Book about Female Doctors?

An unmistakable trend in medical schools across Canada over the past decade has been a steady increase in the percentage of women enrolled. Until the early 1980s, women made up less than one-third of the annual enrolment in Canadian faculties of medicine. Since 1982, however, the number of women enrolling in Canadian medical schools has consistently increased. By 1995, women made up half of those entering medical classes across the country. Since that year, women have been the majority in medical school classes in Canada. Although the high of a 59.1% female incoming cohort across Canada in 2004 has not recurred, the ratio of 55:45 female to male has now become the new normal, with some provinces and territories consistently showing even higher proportions of female students in their intake.

What does this mean for the practice of medicine in Canada? Is it at all of consequence that women are entering and eventually practising medicine in far greater numbers than has ever been seen? The answer is clearly yes, but whether the impact will be positive or negative is yet to be determined. What is clear is that it is past time to consider the implications of these changing demographics in Canadian medicine.

The intent of this book is to explore multiple aspects of women in medicine: how systems, practices, and individuals may or must change as medicine becomes a female-dominated profession. Our medical education is structured based on a system that has always been designed by and for men; this is also true of our health care systems. Issues such as work hours, caregiving, and doctor-patient relationships will all be affected as the ratio of practising physicians shifts from mostly male to mostly female.

In shaping this book, we searched widely for writers and physicians whose recent publications reflected on the current situation, and all the articles included here were in response to direct appeals to our colleagues. Hence, the book encompasses a diverse collection of authors who examine different aspects of the female experience in the profession of medicine. Some of our authors take an academic look at issues such as the history of women in medicine, while other authors present more personal perspectives on aspects of work-life balance and the experiences of women who are trying to navigate a system that was established to suit a male approach. Our authors clearly demonstrate that there is a specific female experience in medicine, and it is very often different from that of their male colleagues. These differences result in changes in how women practise, what type of medicine they choose to practise, and how they want to balance their personal lives with their work.

Our intent with this book is to open a conversation about whether medical education, health systems, and expectations of practice need to be reconsidered in light of the changing face of medicine: from a predominantly male countenance to a more varied and female-driven profession. Because of the shifts underway in medicine, we know this can be no more than the beginning of many such analyses in the years ahead. Yet we hope that this book will provide some of the measurements necessary to understand an important dimension of the profession.

A number of people have assisted us in compiling this book: first, our contributors who often worked against career demands in meeting our deadlines; second, our colleagues across Canada who provided us with suggestions and helpful leads on scholars' works; third, the former chair of the Department of Family Medicine at the University of Alberta, Dr Rick Spooner, who encouraged us to undertake this project despite the fact that most medical writing focuses on short articles, not book-length studies; and finally, our colleagues in family medicine who argued that the book is necessary for young people considering a career in medicine today.

Earle Waugh, Shelley Ross, and Shirley Schipper

Acknowledgments

We wish to acknowledge several people who made this book possible.

Financial support to initiate this volume was provided by the Northern Alberta Family Medicine Academic Enhancement Fund, from the Department of Family Medicine at the University of Alberta. This fund also contributed towards publication of the finished work.

Jenny Wanas contributed the initial literature review that highlighted the issues we wanted to address in this book.

Ipstisam Alexanders, our faithful assistant, kept us on task and handled editing issues with skill and seemingly without end.

Dr L Dujon read an earlier version and provided thoughtful comment.

Our colleagues in family medicine added important ideas in the earlier stages.

FEMALE DOCTORS IN CANADA

Experience and Culture

SECTION ONE

Introductory Perspectives: Female Doctors in Canada

In Canada, there is a national health care system (medicare). This publicly funded, single-payer system was established in 1966 with the passing of the Medical Care Act. Health care is regulated, operated, and funded within each province and territory. Doctors bill the province or territory for each service provided to their patients, and rates are negotiated between the provincial or territorial authority and the doctors' association. Medicare covers only a basic number of services; patients must arrange to pay for those procedures not part of the provincial or territorial plan. Some aspects of care, such as costs associated with home and dental care, eye glasses, and in most cases prescription pharmaceuticals, are the personal responsibility of the patient. The Canada Health Act governs the relationship of the physician to the system, and each province and territory operates its health care system according to its own priorities. Federal funding for special initiatives also plays a role in the care provided; for example, mental health care is provided under other programs, and special funding arrangements may be available for lower income families, depending upon the province or territory. Medicare is gender neutral in its allocations for health care personnel, leaving staffing policy issues to the provinces and territories, so a gender preference in physician is entirely up to the patient. Hospitals generally employ a gender-neutral staffing perspective in keeping with the mores of Canadians.

In this section, the authors address the ways in which the gender-neutral staffing approach affects female doctors in Canada, along with the implications for patient care and career options for women who have chosen to work in medicine. Although Canada's universal health care system does result in some unique policy implications, the rise in numbers of female doctors across North America, the United Kingdom, and Europe means that female doctors in many countries will be facing similar issues, as will the systems in which they operate. Chapter 1 deals specifically with the impact of the recent rise in the number of female doctors on the health care system and provides a basic framework for the focus of this book. Chapter 2 provides a historical scan of women in medicine in Canada through until the late 1990s. Chapter 3 presents an academic overview of the issues arising from the interaction of the feminization of medicine and traditional medical culture, and Chapter 4 outlines the statistics demonstrating how gender differences have modified the health care environment.

1 The Feminization of Medicine: Issues and Implications

SHELLEY ROSS

Both sex – the biological aspects of being female or male – and gender – the cultural roles and meanings ascribed to each sex – are determinants of health. Medical education, research and practice have all suffered from lack of attention to gender and a limited awareness of the effects of the sex-role stereotypes prevalent in our society.

Zelek, Phillips, & Lefebvre, 1997

It is pertinent to ask, 20 years after the observation by Zelek et al. (1997) in a key Canadian medical journal, why we should address again the fundamentals so succinctly expressed therein? Why bother? Have they not been analysed from every perspective since the advent of the social theory of feminism?

The answer to that is both yes and no. Although it is obvious that there has been a sea-change in medical education, there is little indication that equitable upwardly mobile career paths are available or used by women physicians. Moreover, where there is no doubt about technical analyses concerning women's careers in medicine, there have been sparse attempts to convey the *experience* that women have when they enter the profession. That is, numerical evaluations may portray the state of the field, and show parity in some areas, but numerical analysis does not portray the cultural dimensions of being female and being a physician. The assumption is apparent: both males and females will experience the entrance, curricula, process, opportunities, and lifestyle in the same manner.

Several of the articles in this book challenge this assumption. If the assumption is proven suspect, then a host of ethical, policy, and personal issues arise, with major implications for future research: Is the medical profession in Canada on the cusp of fundamental change if the profession increasingly becomes female in the years ahead? What will that mean for medical education, university development, health care planning, delivery of services, and leadership?

Then the reader might enquire, Why just Canada? One can argue that the shifts underway cut across countries and boundaries, so, for example, the glass ceiling seems as prevalent in Britain and Canada as it is evident in the United States. The answer is that Canada's multicultural policy has ramifications for medical education and for the culture of medical delivery. Given the strong role the policy has played since the 1970s in Canada's immigration strategy, it is of great significance. At the very least the issue of integrating international medical graduates into the medical team has seen various degrees of success. Is this because of systemic problems or is it tied to Canadian social differentiation?

These and other related questions are the subject of this volume. By way of engaging the topic, salient background materials need to be provided. These materials are gathered under the following themes:

1. The context: changing demographics in the Canadian health care workforce
2. Canadian medical education: a socializing force for female physicians
3. Career experiences of female physicians and work-life balance
4. Contemporary perspectives on women in medicine
5. Some final considerations that influence the experiences of women in medicine

While clearly there are other issues that could be explored here, these themes provide a foundation for ongoing research into the multiple implications of and for women in medicine. Further, these themes provide a backdrop for the authors who address key contemporary perceptions and share experiences from their perspectives of being women in healthcare professions.

1. The Context: Changing Demographics in the Canadian Health Care Workforce

There has been a steady increase in the number of female students enrolled in medical school over the last 20 years and a subsequent increase in the number of practising female physicians. According to the 2017 *Canadian Medical Education Statistics* report (Association of Faculties of Medicine of Canada, 2017), the proportion of female students has increased from 30% of first-year medical enrolments in the 1980s to the current level of over 50%. Male physicians currently outnumber female physicians almost 2 to 1 (41,379 versus 20,646; Canadian Institute for Health Information, 2007). However, the vast majority of male physicians are ages 40 and older. Female physicians make up two-thirds of practising physicians under the age of 30. This means that as currently practising physicians reach retirement age and leave the profession, the proportion of female practising physicians will increasingly rise.

Why would this demographic shift matter to the average Canadian? The Canadian health care system is faced with several challenges, foremost a need to meet the increasing demands for health care providers. As female students outnumber male students, health care planners need to plan for a shift in how medicine is practised in Canada. A growing body of research finds that female physicians may not follow a traditional model of medical practice. This has direct implications for human health resources, the highest priority area of concern to decision makers according to CIHR's Institute of Health Services and Policy Research in its document that identifies key research areas, *Listening for Direction III* (Law et al., 2008).

Why is this demographic shift so important to Canadian health care planners? Several implications directly affect access to appropriate care and planning for succession. While there is no concern about differences in *quality* of care between male and female physicians, research findings suggest health care planners do need to account for differences in *quantity* of care provided when planning for succession in the health care workforce:

- Female physicians under 31 years of age, and those ages 46 to 50, provided significantly fewer services (at least 21% fewer) than their male counterparts (Constant & Léger, 2008).
- At all ages, female physicians do not reach parity with male physicians in the services they provide (Constant & Léger, 2008).
- As the proportion of female practising physicians increasingly rises, there will be a concurrent decrease in the total quantity of services provided (Constant & Léger, 2008).
- Controlling for demographic and other characteristics, female physicians retire 4.1 years earlier than their male counterparts (Hedden et al., 2017).

- Female physicians are more likely than male physicians to
  - prematurely leave the practice of medicine permanently or leave practice temporarily for stress leave (Simon, 1986)
  - experience burn-out (McMurray et al., 2000)
  - commit suicide (Schernhammer & Colditz, 2004)

A further difference between female and male physicians exists in the choice of specialty. Female doctors are more likely than males to choose family medicine and less likely to choose surgical specialties, based on recent data from the Canadian Post-MD Education Registry (2016). When female post-MDs do choose surgical specialties, they are more likely to choose obstetrics/gynecology than any other surgical specialty. As Canada's aging population of surgical specialists retires, there are fewer new specialists to replace them, creating an issue of succession and access to appropriate care for health care planners.

In her chapter on the history of women doctors in Canada, Heather Stanley explores in detail the issues that women in medicine have faced since before formal medical education began in Canada. Stanley also chronicles changes in systems and assumptions about the roles of women in caring for the ill as medicine transformed as a profession. Of particular interest is the way in which the professionalization of medicine was accompanied by a drastically different view of the acceptability of women as students and practitioners of medicine. This historical overview sets the tone for the remainder of this volume by placing the "new wave" of feminization of medicine in a historical context.

Surprisingly, despite the evidence-based reasons that the feminization of medicine requires a closer look from educators, policymakers, and health care planners, this area has been either overlooked or dismissed as a non-issue. Raising the topic of the feminization of medicine often sparks a defensive reaction from both men and women: in a society where we strive for equity, it is seen as equally offensive to suggest that women (1) have different experiences in their journeys to becoming healthcare professionals, and (2) will demonstrate different practice patterns as a result of those experiences. Both men and women insist that healthcare professions – particularly the profession of being a physician – are gender-/sex-blind. Indeed, the very claim of neutrality is not value-free: Tsikata's article underlines the fact that medicine has a particular *culture*, that it is deeply embedded in both the perceptions of Canadians and the assumptions that practitioners have, and that this plays a role in the entire system. As will be seen throughout this book, both objective research and personal experiences call into question many of the assumptions in this structure. Finally, Hamza and Ross offer an objective view of the changing demographics of the medical profession through a presentation of the statistics from a variety of databases.

2. Canadian Medical Education: A Socializing Force for Female Physicians

Throughout this volume, the female physicians who contributed chapters (Bethune, Schabort, Ross, Dollin, Gartke, Gautam, Kernaghan, Tsikata, and Feldman) have included some personal stories of their experiences in Canadian medical education. These experiences are often framed further within an exploration of research and policy that affect female medical students and residents as they pursue training. Pertinent to this theme of the socializing force of education, Bethune's chapter addresses the issues of gendered experiences in medical school and the hidden curriculum around women in medicine. Although medical education has changed fundamentally since the early days in the 1860s, there are still surprising elements in the hidden curriculum that affect female trainees differently than their male colleagues.

Early pioneers – those women who dared to challenge the male status quo and pursue studies in medicine – faced the prevailing attitude of "monstrous brains and puny bodies" that was influenced by religious norms and social values in 1873 (Creek, 2007). During this time, women were seen as susceptible to both physical and mental disorders and therefore deemed not fit for the medical profession (Creek, 2007).

Dr Jenny Kidd Trout and Dr Emily Stowe both faced intense obstacles in attempting to pursue medical education in Canada; both were forced to complete part of their education in the United States before becoming the first and second (respectively) licensed female physicians in Canada. It was due to Emily Stowe's tremendous pressures on the University of Toronto that her daughter Augusta Stowe-Gullen was permitted entry into the field of medicine (Creek, 2007; Collections Canada, 2008).

Despite Stowe's efforts, Creek (2007) and other scholars note that throughout the nineteenth century women's role in medicine remained relegated to that of a patient. Duffin and Stuart's (2012) research demonstrates how women's role in feminizing medicine meant more rights for women at large especially in terms of reproductive rights, control of family size, and increased power for women in the workplace.

While medical education and societal pressures have changed considerably from Trout and Stowe's era, the need to pay attention to women's educational experiences is essential to understanding the changing medical culture or feminization of medicine. Despite increasing numbers of women in fields of medicine since the nineteenth and twentieth centuries, barriers still exist for female medical students and doctors within medical education, policy, and practice. The Canadian Institute for Health Information (2010; Buske, 2013) estimates that the number and ratio of physicians to patients has been increasing, with a concurrent increase in the numbers of female physicians. While socio-historical milestones on the Canadian macro national and global levels are often notable in terms of advances for women within medicine and medical education, as previously described, some scholars note that these are not always beneficial or helpful. Indeed, they argue, gender bias still permeates medical education and its educators through socialization on the psychological, familial, cultural, educational, and societal levels (Candib, 2006; Phillips, 1995). Nevertheless, Martin, Arnold, and Parker (1988) describe how the feminist movement during the 1960s was essential in paving the way for a rise in female medical graduates that occurred since that time. From the 1960s onwards, 5% of all medical graduates were women, but this was a number that remained steady for 50 years (Martin et al., 1988).

Examples of how women physicians continue to encounter barriers within medical education are numerous within the research. When entering non-traditional male-dominated fields, such as surgery, research suggests that women medical students may not persist to graduation because certain fields are perceived as "unwelcoming," with a dearth of female role models and the existence of sexual harassment (Borges et al., 2012; Komaromy et al., 1993; Crutcher et al., 2011). The reasons how and why medical students choose to enter certain medical fields, according to the British Columbia Medical Association (2011), need to be better understood to better align medical educational policy. For example, despite the fact that women compose 50% of medical students, they only occupy 16% of gastroenterology fellowships in the United States, and throughout the fellowship years, their numbers steadily decline (Burke et al., 2005). Currently, Gradstein (2008) argues that women residents are able to benefit more from education and balance it with parenting pressures while medical undergraduates do not. Better alignment of medical policy and education is therefore needed to prevent unnecessary expenditure on physician training and education

(Bates et al., 2008; British Columbia Medical Association, 2011; Embriaco et al., 2012).

A further consideration in examining medical education and women's experiences is presented in Inge Schabort's chapter. Schabort looks specifically at the experiences of female international medical graduates (IMG) – those who completed their medical school training outside Canada. Schabort discusses the experiences of both non-Canadians who want to practise in Canada and Canadians who attended medical school outside Canada and want to return home for postgraduate training. Female IMGs face all the same issues in their training in Canada as do female trainees and physicians who completed all their training in Canada; however, female IMGs face even more challenges, including increased financial burden (especially for Canadians who train abroad), increased stress in pursuing sometimes overwhelming or burdensome processes to achieve licensure, and cultural issues that can become serious obstacles to their quality of life.

3. Career Experiences of Female Physicians in Medicine and Work-Life Balance

As discussed, women's career choices are influenced by their educational socialization. With respect to career choices of women in medicine, scholars point to various influencing factors, such as female role models within educational spheres and the need for women to consider work and family balance to a greater degree than their male contemporaries (Viscomi et al., 2013). The absence of female role models within medical fields affects socialization of women into specific feminine medical fields (Malicki, 2007). Heather Stanley's chapter includes an overview of the evolving historical pressures that women have faced in making career choices.

The enduring "femininity" of certain fields despite the apparent and ongoing changes in traditional norms and societal values in Canada asks whether or not the medical field has kept up or lags behind a post-feminist era. Research (Scott et al., 2010) within obstetrics and gynecology specializations notes that the most significant predictor of career choice is being female, as opposed to any other factor, such as being younger, having parents in the field, or growing up in a large town. Malicki (2007) concurs with Scott and colleagues, stating that obstetrics and gynecology remains the field with the highest percentage of women at 71%, followed by pediatrics at 67%. Moreover, women who succeed in male-dominated fields, such as orthopedic surgery, feel as if they are maligned or punished for it. Malicki (2007) states, "Women who behave in ways typically reserved for men are found to be less socially appealing than men who behave similarly or women who behave more in line with normative prescriptions" (p. 2). Interestingly, the research finds that men who enter a field that is considered feminine will similarly experience social exclusion. The impact of female physician success within male dominated fields across age groups and college majors is, according to Malicki, important to consider for future research, given that women are entering male-dominated fields of medicine in higher numbers. Indeed, females outnumber males in fields such as family medicine, pediatrics, geriatrics, endocrinology, and medical genetics (Biringer & Carroll, 2012).

As women progress through the stages of their medical education, their decisions are influenced by different factors from those considered by their male counterparts. Women considering a career in surgery often believe their family life would be subsumed by it, and therefore some decline the career path after starting it (Mobilos et al., 2008). By contrast, male physicians enter various fields in medicine with comparatively less decision making stress than females regarding how specialization would impact their family life (Mobilos et al., 2008). Scott et al. (2008) similarly found an overall downward trend in enrolment by medical students in surgery in terms of those who not only had a "surgical personality" but also shared several common demographic characteristics, such as being younger, being single, having university-educated parents, and living in urban areas (p. 373). Medical students who selected a career in surgery were more dedicated to a "hospital vs. social orientation" (p. 375). Scott et al. (2008) argue that because of the increasing number of women entering medicine overall, surgical medical education must begin to reflect the norms and values of this feminization trend. According to Scott and colleagues, this can be accomplished by beginning to update educational policies that embrace the entrance of women in schools of surgery and by overtly attempting to rectify some of the barriers women perceive. Regarding quality of life and the stress endured by females practising medicine, scholars contend that, for the most part, women physicians make most of the decisions related to family life, which in turn negatively affects their quality of life and results in more stress related to work than male physicians experience. This has remained an enduring aspect regardless of the increasing numbers of women in medical practice. Thus it is argued throughout the literature that medical education, practice, and policies are experienced and lived differently by female physicians, and therefore attention needs to be paid to female physicians' psychological, familial, and career experiences. These experiences have an impact not only on the physicians themselves but also on their families, and on the patients they serve. Rectifying this situation will benefit quality of service for all Canadians.

The chapter by Shelley Ross accurately reflects how medicine is lived and experienced differently by women than by their male colleagues. Through a combination of sharing her personal experiences as a female family physician and providing a review of the literature, Ross presents evidence for the differences between men and women in attaining an acceptable work-life balance as physicians. As noted above, Schabort elaborates on the information presented by Ross by adding the extra layer of stresses experienced by female IMG physicians.

Kathleen Gartke presents in detail the multiple factors that influence career trajectories for women, including systems issues and pressures from society, family, and policymakers. She explores how generational differences have and continue to affect female physicians, from how experienced female mentors offer advice to being compared to older male colleagues in terms of hours worked and types of practice that modern female physicians are willing to establish.

Female physicians often encounter inequity during medical education in various forms, such as intimidation, harassment, and discrimination (Crutcher et al., 2011). This trend continues throughout their careers, manifesting as unwanted attention, verbal abuse, and harassment (Farber et al., 2000). For example, female physicians practising general internal medicine were more likely to discharge patients for "sexually explicit language," "personal questions," and "overly affectionate language" (Farber et al., 2000). Minor transgressions include actions such as gift-giving; however, the most serious ones include sexual behaviours and physical abuse. According to Miedema et al. (2010), female physicians also encounter abuse from co-workers, thereby demonstrating that negative experiences may not only come from patients. In the latter case, the victim is usually a female physician and the offender is most often a male (Miedema et al., 2010).

Female physicians often lack the role models to enter and remain within male-dominated fields of medical education and internships. However, when women are in medical education, their presence has been positively associated with supportive career guidance and constructive steps toward changing gender policies and therefore enhancing the educational aspirations of female medical students and residents (Borges et al., 2012). Research during the 1990s suggested that there was resistance to women entering academic medicine, that such institutions are male dominated, and that they are considered "old boys" networks (Lent et al., 2007; Leopando, 2002). The notion of a glass ceiling within medical education and leadership fields of practice, pay, and research is still a dominant stream within much of the research on the feminization of medicine. The chapter by Cheri Bethune includes personal experiences of the challenges of academic medicine for women, and Shelley Ross and Monica Olsen offer insights into how female physicians respond to women in leadership positions.

Compounding female physicians' experiences of career-related stress is the fact that for the most part, female physicians are also the primary caregivers at home. Role conflict is a major source of burnout for female physicians in their relationships and marriages (Shanafelt et al., 2012). This is supplemented with research among male and female physicians in Newfoundland and Labrador that found that although male physicians felt a sense of guilt when they did not engage in many child-rearing activities, they were not assumed or expected to "naturally do so" (Parsons et al., 2009). One of the most enduring factors that aids in protecting physician relationships with their spouses, regardless of medical practice specialization, has been found to be the time that physicians set aside for their families (Shanafelt et al., 2012).

Verlander (2004) explored the conundrum that female physicians face regarding when and whether to bear children, as well as how much time to spend with their families. This research found that male physicians do not experience these decisions to the same extent nor with the same consequences. For example, Verlander notes that the "most opportune" time for a woman to biologically have children is also the most demanding time occupationally. Verlander's research has even found that female doctors and medical students timed their pregnancies for the most opportune career times: after completion of training, during residency, and in third year of medical school. Because women bear children and are often the ones linked to child rearing, they must often take breaks from work responsibilities, a fact that their colleagues may resent (Verlander).

Discussion of burnout is important, since not all female physicians experience depression, burnout, or substance abuse at the same rate or at the same levels. In addition, the stigma regarding depression and substance abuse among colleagues and society make these issues difficult to discuss. Research illustrates that female physicians' experiences may vary by the medical specialization in which female physicians practice. Experience of depression and substance abuse as a result of burnout and role overload is reported in the literature. Research has examined how the demands on women in domestic and career spheres adversely impact their psychological health through burnout, contributing to depression and substance abuse.

Female physicians dealing with severely ill patients, such as in medical emergency and critical care, experience higher levels of burnout because of the higher stress inherent in those specialties in comparison to obstetrics and gynecology, internal medicine, and family medicine. The ability to balance career-related stress and avoid burnout or depression in occupations such as emergency medicine and critical care is positively related to physician self-care (Embriaco et al., 2012; Trollope-Kumar, 2012). Female physicians' experience with depression is higher than that of male physicians and of the general female population, illustrating a need for policymakers to pay attention to the consequences of the feminization of medicine (Bowman & Gross, 1990).

4. Contemporary Perspectives on Women in Medicine

The nature of gendered education and practice has raised questions regarding the specific nature of gendered dialogue with patients and the impacts this has on medical delivery services and practices. Female physicians communicate differently with their patients than do male physicians, and to an extent researchers debate how this differentially influences the nature of medical practice, such as screening and counselling patients. This topic appears throughout the chapters of this book. Erin Fredericks examines practice style and communication differences through the lens of female physicians as ethical decision makers and explores how men and women differ in how they arrive at decisions, how they consider evidence, and how physicians communicate those decisions to their patients. Perle Feldman shares some personal experiences in practice style and ways of approaching different aspects of practice. Monica Olsen and colleagues offer an overview of how practice styles have changed or need to change. They offer recommendations to policymakers that would improve opportunities for women to create practice styles that work best for them and to ensure quality patient care and appropriate work-life balance for female physicians.

Some of the changes already seen in how medicine is practised – sharing call, taking a more patient-centred approach – reflect the subtle influence that female physicians have had on the profession.

Various factors in addition to the gender of the physician affect gendered communication between patients and physicians, including physician-patient gender pairings, rural-urban settings, and the training of physicians. Some research has demonstrated that female physicians communicate differently when screening for breast cancer and are more likely to offer screening mammography than are male physicians (Meguerditchian et al., 2012). However, the research cautions that findings regarding screening mammography are higher within rural settings where patients are more likely to continuously visit the same doctor and where patients encounter more barriers (Meguerditchian et al., 2012). Meguerditchian and colleagues' findings corroborate these breast cancer screening claims and state that the communication skills of male physicians who were found not to screen females may be made up for through more targeted training of male physicians.

There are claims that female physicians are more likely to be both emotionally focused and patient-centred. According to a systematic review by Roter et al. (2002) female physicians were more likely to engage in patient-centred counselling and emotional positive talk. Roter and colleagues' research examined and analysed 23 observational study databases. The only medical specialty in which males were found to spend comparatively more time than female physicians was obstetrics and gynecology. Conversely, research by Bertakis et al. (2009) suggests that physician gender is not the only characteristic affecting physician-patient communication; factors such as physician-patient gender concordance are necessary to consider as well. Although physicians engage in patient-centred communication with their female patients, female patients behave and communicate differently than male patients, and this in itself is a contributing factor to patient-doctor communication and interaction (Bertakis et al., 2009).

5. Some Final Considerations That Influence the Experiences of Women in Medicine

Geographical Location, Compensation, and Assumptions of Working Less

Geographical location, that is, rural versus urban, is a variable identified by research as one that influences the way in which medicine is practised. It is thus worth examining the different dynamics and pressures on female physicians in these settings. As mentioned previously, the communication patterns of female physicians vary in rural and urban settings. Other variables that are sensitive to geographic location are patient-physician boundaries, physician work-life balance, and the nature of patient expectations.

A large scale survey study of Canadian physicians conducted by Miedema and colleagues (2010) found that physicians working in inner cities, small towns, or rural communities were more likely to experience instances of severe abuse by patients or patients' families than were physicians who worked in urban or suburban settings. Buske (2013) documented how 55% of female physicians working in rural areas are younger than 45 years of age, compared with 45% of women in the same age group in the urban areas. According to Buske, rural family physicians work more hours yet report being more satisfied than their urban counterparts. This was attributed to the ability of rural physicians to balance their workload and personal life. Conversely, Incitti et al. (2003) found that female physicians in rural areas work longer hours and are less satisfied than male physicians in rural areas and also less satisfied than male and female physicians in urban areas. Similar findings arose in comparative research examining Australia and Canada by Viscomi et al. (2013). These findings suggest that there needs to be better training for both recruitment and retention of physicians in rural areas. The fact that there are conflicting findings regarding satisfaction of women in rural areas points to the need for more research in this area.

Concerning medical practice and pay, women in all fields of medicine still seem to encounter the notion that they must prove themselves; even when they do succeed by completing medical school and entering their chosen medical field, they do not seem to be financially rewarded to the same extent as men. Chen and Chevalier (2012) note that female primary care physicians still do not receive a return on investment for the many years they put into medical education. Moreover, whereas salaries may be greater than in other specialties, such as surgery, women are sparsely represented in these male-dominated areas, and there is a lack of mentorship (Chen & Chevalier, 2012; Zhuge et al., 2011). Chen and Cavalier also believe that part of the problem with the lack of a return on investment experienced by women is the fact that female physicians overestimate how many hours they will actually be working. For these researchers, therefore, not only would female physicians have made a better "choice on investment" had they chosen a physician-assistant occupation but they would also have had a better work-life balance. Similar research in the United States finds that female physicians earn $22,000 less than males; endure greater job complexity, such as having female patients who present more complex psychosocial problems; and have less control over their work schedules (McMurray et al., 2000).

Instead of examining the micro, meso, and macro system levels of hardships that women physicians have had to endure and overcome to become doctors, there are those who continue to place blame on women physicians themselves. Duffin and Stuart (2012) cite an example of a *Globe and Mail* pundit who, contrary to Canadian medical deans' evidence, blamed women physicians for doctor shortages. Ross (2003) states that the feminization of the medical profession is creating a pink-collar profession and that by 2020 women will outnumber men. However, she notes that despite the feminization of medicine, the glass ceiling persists and pay inequities remain. She attributes these to the specialties women physicians select and to the need to accommodate women's work-life balance in education, training, residency, and practice. Changes to accommodate women's needs in work-life balance benefits female physicians and their families (Ross, 2003). Within academic medicine and educational research, Wenger and Lave (2008) contend there is a need for more women in leadership positions within meso-level academic institutions, such as editorial review boards to represent issues of concern to women in scientific medical research.

This volume addresses many of the issues raised in this exposition, and our authors have attempted to portray precisely how women in medicine perceive themselves in contemporary Canada. They provide a rich tapestry of approaches and styles in their writing, reflecting the multidimensional situation that they experience. Consequently, we begin with Heather Stanley's overview in **"Unsex Me Here!" Gender as a Barrier to Female Practice: A Historical Introduction to Women Doctors in Canada,** with insights into women in medicine from 1865 to today, and then move to Setorme Tsikata's academic examination of the **Cultural Barriers within Medicine** itself. Hamza and Ross give perspective to the issues discussed in the first three chapters of this volume by offering an objective overview of the **Current State of Women in Medicine: The Statistics.**

In Section 2 of this book, two chapters present some of the issues and challenges facing women as they progress through the education system and out into their careers: Cheri Bethune examines the educational hindrances and the career sequelae of those experiences in **Gendered Experience, Role Models and Mentorship, Leadership, and the**

Hidden Curriculum, while Inge Schabort offers insight into the extra challenges faced by women from abroad who have to navigate the same challenges as Canadian-trained female physicians while also trying to adapt to a medical culture that places them at an added disadvantage in her chapter on **Female International Medical Graduates in Canada**.

In Section 3 on the career experiences of women in medicine, Kathleen Garke and Janet Dollin offer an experiential assessment of the forces and barriers on women in their **Career Trajectory of Women in Medicine**. This is followed by Shelley Ross's account of her personal journey through medical practice and leadership in medicine as she also navigated **Quality of Life/Life-Work Balance**.

In Section 4 on contemporary perspectives of women in medicine, our authors portray the complexity women face in this career. Erin Fredericks sketches the unique experiences of women in her chapter addressing **Women Physicians as Ethical Decision Makers**, while Monica Olsen, Mamta Gautam, and Gillian Kernaghan present the challenges women face while engaging in a career option that is itself constantly shifting in their contribution, **Women and New Forms of Medicine**. This section is rounded out by the contribution of Perle Feldman, a personal account of her experiences as a female physician practising across a span of years that have seen large-scale changes, in her chapter **Patients, Women Family Doctors, and Patient-Centred Care**.

The engagement with these writers provides important access to the situation women in medicine face in Canada today. Our final chapter in Section 5 summarizes many of the issues raised by our authors and offers both possible solutions and areas where more research is needed to ensure that the feminization of medicine is a positive advancement to health care, both at the systems level and (most importantly) at the patient-care level.

REFERENCES

Association of Faculties of Medicine of Canada. (2017). *Canadian medical education statistics, 2017.* Ottawa, Canada: Author.

Bates, J., Lovato, C., & Buller-Taylor, T. (2008). "Mind the gap": Seven key issues in aligning medical education and healthcare policy. *Healthcare Policy, 4*(2), 46–58. Retrieved from https://www.ncbi.nlm.nih.gov/pmc/articles/PMC2645211/ Medline:19377369

Bertakis, K.D., Franks, P., & Epstein, R.M. (2009). Patient-centered communication in primary care: Physician and patient gender and gender concordance. *Journal of Women's Health (2002)*, *18*(4), 539–45. https://doi.org/10.1089/jwh.2008.0969 Medline:19361322

Biringer, A., & Carroll, J.C. (2012). What does the feminization of family medicine mean? *CMAJ*, *184*(15), 1752. https://doi.org/10.1503/cmaj.120771 Medline:23008491

Bowman, M., & Gross, M.L. (1990) Overview of research on women in medicine: Issues for policymakers. In W.G. Rothstein (Ed.), *Readings in American health care* (pp. 190–8). Madison: University of Wisconsin Press.

Borges, N.J., Navarro, A.M., & Grover, A.C. (2012). Women physicians: Choosing a career in academic medicine. *Academic Medicine: Journal of the Association of American Medical Colleges*, *87*(1), 105–14. https://doi.org/10.1097/ACM.0b013e31823ab4a8 Medline:22104052

British Columbia Medical Association. (2011). *Doctors today and tomorrow: Planning British Columbia's physician workforce*. Vancouver, Canada: Author.

Burke, C., Sastri, S., Jacobsen, G., Arlow, F., Karlstadt, R., & Raymond, P. (2005). Gender disparity in the practice of gastroenterology: The first 5 years of a career. *The American Journal of Gastroenterology*, *100*, 259–64. https://doi.org/10.1111/j.1572-0241.2005.41005.x

Buske, L. (2013). First practice: Family physicians initially locating in rural areas. *Canadian Journal of Rural Medicine: The Official Journal of the Society of Rural Physicians of Canada*, *18*(3), 80–5. Medline:23806431

Canadian Institute for Health Information. (2007). *Health indicators, 2007.* Ottawa, Canada: Author.

Canadian Institute for Health Information. (2010). *Supply, distribution, and migration of Canadian physicians, 2009*. Ottawa, Canada: Author.

Candib, L.M. (2006, Sep-Oct). Si, doctora. *Annals of Family Medicine*, *4*(5), 460–2. https://doi.org/10.1370/afm.572 Medline:17003149

Canadian Post-MD Education Registry. (2016). Fact sheet: Gender trends in Canadian postgraduate medical training. Retrieved from https://caper.ca/en/news/fact-sheet-on-gender-in-canadian-post-md-training/

Chen, M., & Chevalier, J. (2012). Are women overinvesting in education? Evidence from the medical profession. *Journal of Human Capital*, *6*(2), 124–49. https://doi.org/10.1086/665536

Collections Canada. (2008). Dr. Emily Howard Stowe. Retrieved from http://www.collectionscanada.gc.ca/physicians/030002-2500-e.html

Constant, A., & Léger, P.T. (2008). Estimating differences between male and female physician service provision using panel data. *Health Economics*, *17*(11), 1295–315. https://doi.org/10.1002/hec.1344 Medline:18404663

Creek, K. (2007). *Proceedings from the 16th Annual History of Medicine Days: Monstrous brains and puny bodies: The struggle for female physicians in Canada, 1800–1950*. Winnipeg: University of Manitoba.

Crutcher, R.A., Szafran, O., Woloschuk, W., Chatur, F., & Hansen, C. (2011). Family medicine graduates' perceptions of intimidation, harassment, and discrimination during residency training. *BMC Medical Education, 11*(1), 88. https://doi.org/10.1186/1472-6920-11-88 Medline:22018090

Duffin, J., & Stuart, M. (2012). Feminization of Canadian medicine: voices from the second wave. *Canadian Bulletin of Medical History, 29*(1), 83–100. https://doi.org/10.3138/cbmh.29.1.83 Medline:22849252

Embriaco, N., Hraiech, S., Azoulay, E., Baumstarck-Barrau, K., Forel, J.M., Kentish-Barnes, N., …, & Papazian, L. (2012). Symptoms of depression in ICU physicians. *Annals of Intensive Care, 2*(1), 34. https://doi.org/10.1186/2110-5820-2-34 Medline:22839744

Farber, N.J., Novack, D.H., Silverstein, J., Davis, E.B., Weiner, J., & Boyer, E.G. (2000, Nov). Physicians' experiences with patients who transgress boundaries. *Journal of General Internal Medicine, 15*(11), 770–5. https://doi.org/10.1046/j.1525-1497.2000.90734.x Medline:11119168

Gradstein, M. (2008). Mothering in education: Parenting policies in medical education. *Atlantis* (Wolfville, NS), *32*(2), 149–56.

Hedden, L., Lavergne, M.R., McGrail, K.M., Law, M.R., Cheng, L., Ahuja, M.A., & Barer, M.L. (2017). Patterns of physician retirement and preretirement activity: A population-based cohort study. *Canadian Medical Association Journal, 189*(49), E1517–23. https://doi.org/10.1503/cmaj.170231 Medline:29229713

Incitti, F., Rourke, J., Rourke, L.L., & Kennard, M. (2003). Rural women family physicians. Are they unique? *Canadian Family Physician, 49*, 320–7. Medline:12675545

Komaromy, M., Bindman, A.B., Haber, R.J., & Sande, M.A. (1993, Feb 4). Sexual harassment in medical training. *The New England Journal of Medicine, 328*(5), 322–6. https://doi.org/10.1056/NEJM199302043280507 Medline:8419819

Law, S., Flood, C., & Gagnon, D. (2008). Listening for direction III: National consultation on health services and policy issues: 2007–2010. Retrieved from https://www.cfhi-fcass.ca/PublicationsAndResources/ResourcesAndTools/ListeningForDirection.aspx

Lent, B., & Wonca Working Party on Women Family Medicine. (2007). Gender equity: Canadian contribution to international initiative. *Canadian Family Physician, 53*(3), 488–90. Medline:17872687

Leopando, Z.E. (2002). Championing family medicine—Regional Wonca growth toward maturity. *Asia Pacific Family Medicine, 1*(1), 5–6. Retrieved from http://www.apfmj-archive.com/afm1.1/afm_008.pdf. https://doi.org/10.1046/j.1444-1683.2002.00008.x

Malicki, M. (2007). Code blue! (Or pink!): Perceptions of men and women physicians in specific gender dominated medical subfields. *UW-L Journal of Undergraduate Research, X*, 1–3.

Martin, S.C., Arnold, R.M., & Parker, R.M. (1988). Gender and medical socialization. *Journal of Health and Social Behavior, 29*(4), 333–43. https://doi.org/10.2307/2136867 Medline:3253324

McMurray, J.E., Linzer, M., Konrad, T.R., Douglas, J., Shugerman, R., Nelson, K., & The SGIM Career Satisfaction Study Group. (2000). The work lives of women physicians: Results from the physician work life study. *Journal of General Internal Medicine, 15*(6), 372–80. https://doi.org/10.1111/j.1525-1497.2000.im9908009.x Medline:10886471

Meguerditchian, A.N., Dauphinee, D., Girard, N., Eguale, T., Riedel, K., Jacques, A., …, & Tamblyn, R. (2012). Do physician communication skills influence screening mammography utilization? *BMC Health Services Research, 12*(1), 219. Retrieved from https://www.biomedcentral.com/1472-6963/12/219. https://doi.org/10.1186/1472-6963-12-219 Medline:22831648

Miedema, B., Hamilton, R., Lambert-Lanning, A., Tatemichi, S.R., Lemire, F., Manca, D., & Ramsden, V.R. (2010). Prevalence of abusive encounters in the workplace of family physicians: A minor, major, or severe problem? *Canadian Family Physician, 56*(3), e101–8.

Mobilos, S., Chan, M., & Brown, J.B. (2008). Women in medicine: The challenge of finding balance. *Canadian Family Physician, 54*(9), 1285–6.e5. Medline:18791106

Parsons, W.L., Duke, P.S., Snow, P., & Edwards, A. (2009). Physicians as parents: Parenting experiences of physicians in Newfoundland and Labrador. *Canadian Family Physician, 55*(8), 808–9.e4. Medline:19675267

Phillips, S. (1995). The social context of women's health: goals and objectives for medical education. *CMAJ, 152*(4), 507–11. Medline:7859198

Ross, S. (2003). The feminization of medicine. *AMA Journal of Ethics, 5*(9). Retrieved from http://virtualmentor.ama-assn.org/2003/09/msoc1-0309.html

Roter, D.L., Hall, J.A., & Aoki, Y. (2002). Physician gender effects in medical communication: a meta-analytic review. *Journal of the American Medical Association, 288*(6), 756–64. https://doi.org/10.1001/jama.288.6.756 Medline:12169083

Schernhammer, E.S., & Colditz, G.A. (2004). Suicide rates among physicians: a quantitative and gender assessment (meta-analysis). *The American Journal of Psychiatry, 161*(12), 2295–302. https://doi.org/10.1176/appi.ajp.161.12.2295 Medline:15569903

Scott, I., Matajcek, B., Gowans, D., Wright, B., & Brenneis, F. (2008). Choosing a career in surgery: Factors that influence Canadian medical students' interests pursuing a surgical career. *Canadian Journal of Medicine, 51*(5), 371–7.

Scott, I.M., Nasmith, T., Gowans, M.C., Wright, B.J., & Brenneis, F.R. (2010). Obstetrics and gynaecology as a career choice: a cohort study of Canadian medical students. *Journal of Obstetrics and Gynaecology Canada, 32*(11), 1063–9. https://doi.org/10.1016/S1701-2163(16)34715-6 Medline:21176319

Shanafelt, T.D., Boone, S., Tan, L., Dyrbye, L.N., Sotile, W., Satele, D., …, & Oreskovich, M.R. (2012). Burnout and satisfaction with work-life balance among US physicians relative to the general US population. *Archives of Internal Medicine, 172*(18), 1377–85. https://doi.org/10.1001/archinternmed.2012.3199 Medline:22911330

Simon, W. (1986). Suicide among physicians: prevention and postvention. *Crisis, 7*(1), 1–13. Medline:3490952

Trollope-Kumar, K. (2012). Do we overdramatize family physician burnout?: NO. *Canadian Family Physician, 58*(7), 731–3, 735–7. Medline:22798458

Verlander, G. (2004). Female physicians: balancing career and family. *Academic Psychiatry: The Journal of the American Association of Directors of Psychiatric Residency Training and the Association for Academic Psychiatry, 28*(4), 331–6. https://doi.org/10.1176/appi.ap.28.4.331 Medline:15673831

Viscomi, M., Larkins, S., & Gupta, T.S. (2013). Recruitment and retention of general practitioners in rural Canada and Australia: a review of the literature. *Canadian Journal of Rural Medicine, 18*(1), 13–23. Medline:23259963

Wenger, E., & Lave, J. (2008). *Situated learning: Legitimate peripheral participation* (18th ed.). New York: Cambridge University Press.

Zelek, B., Phillips, S.P., & Lefebvre, Y. (1997). Gender sensitivity in medical curricula. *CMAJ, 156*(9), 1297–300.

Zhuge, Y., Kaufman, J., Simeone, D.M., Chen, H., & Velazquez, O.C. (2011). Is there still a glass ceiling for women in academic surgery? *Annals of Surgery, 253*(4), 637–43. https://doi.org/10.1097/SLA.0b013e3182111120 Medline:21475000

2 "Unsex Me Here!" Gender as a Barrier to Female Practice: A Historical Introduction to Women Doctors in Canada

HEATHER STANLEY

When, in 1865, local charwoman Mrs Bishop laid out the body of the famed Doctor James Barry in preparation for his burial, she made a shocking discovery. Barry, a noted surgeon, the former inspector-general of hospitals for Upper and Lower Canada, and a decorated medical officer in the British Army, had female genitalia. Later, Mrs Bishop would also claim the body showed evidence that Barry had borne a child.

We know very little about Barry's life, though it seems he[1] was born a female named Miranda Barry sometime in the last years of the eighteenth century. By 1812, he was living as a man and had graduated as a surgeon from Edinburgh University, after which he practised medicine throughout the British Empire, including in Canada, as a member of the British Army. Given his appointment as the inspector-general of hospitals for Upper and Lower Canada, he would have been the first female doctor to practise in the nation (Hacker, 2001). What can we make of such a story?

First, we must acknowledge the prospect that Barry was a transgender man who lived that existence as much as was possible in the time in which he was born. It is also possible that Barry was born as an intersexed infant. Children born with ambiguous genitalia were almost always assigned the female gender at birth because it was thought a greater cruelty to be assigned the male gender and have to live with a

1 Given the possibility that Barry was indeed a transgender man and that he seems to have chosen to live his life as member of the male gender, I have chosen to use the male pronoun to describe him.

very small, and possibly non-procreative, penis (Stanley, 2013). Barry might have then assumed his true gender later in life. This was the conclusion reached by Staff-Surgeon Major McKinnon, who examined Barry's body after Mrs Bishop's revelation. Some historians argue McKinnon was a well-known rival of Barry's and used his posthumous diagnosis of hermaphrodism to defame Barry and undermine his accomplishments (Hacker, 2001). However, it is the last possibility that is of most interest to this work: could it have been that Barry was born a woman and decided that the only way to be a doctor at the height of the Victorian age was to assume a male name and identity?

During the Victorian era medical men were working hard to shed the profession's former classification as largely unskilled manual labour and to replace it with the idea that medicine was a gentleman's profession requiring scientific ability and rational thought. At the same time medical science was firmly entrenched in the long-held, scientifically "proven" paradigm that women were ruled by their reproductive biology, and thus it was inappropriate, and even dangerous, for them to undertake any kind of work requiring masculinized higher orders of thinking (Moscucci, 1990; Mitchinson, 1991; Schiebinger, 1993; Warsh, 2010). When the aspirations of medical men to improve their profession, the scientific views on the female body, and strict Victorian gender roles interwove, they created an Aegean knot that left women who desired to practise medicine very little room to manoeuvre. In fact, any woman practising medicine in the Victorian era was forced to be, by her very nature, a living, breathing paradox as she engaged in the very medical science that proclaimed to the world that she was abnormal. Though the science behind the delegitimization of women outside their roles as wives and mothers changed throughout the twentieth century, the medical image of the female body as mentally and biologically inferior to the male persisted. Medical women during this time would have been torn between their female identity and their desire to be a doctor – identities that society and medicine put in binary opposition. Could it be that Barry, faced with this insurmountable paradox of identity, chose to pass as a man instead? If so, how did other women overcome this social and medical bias to combine their social role as women with their vocation in medicine?

In this historical introduction, the lives of some of the Canadian Famous Firsts – familiar names such as Emily Howard Stowe and Helen MacMurchy – are re-examined with the Victorian (and post-Victorian) binary of woman-doctor in mind to demonstrate both the inequities that kept the numbers of practising female doctors small and the strategies used by these women to gain power within social and medical structures that systematically disadvantaged them. Unlike many previous histories of female medical pioneers, this is not a celebratory story demonstrating a clear upward trajectory from an unfortunate past to a glorious present. That the women profiled in this chapter broke down barriers and challenged stereotypes cannot be denied. That they often did so by exerting their own power over more socially disadvantaged groups – namely poorer or non-white women – also cannot, and should not, be denied. It should also be clear that while the days where medical schools, professional organizations, and hospitals enacted policy to keep the number of women doctors small (or non-existent) have thankfully diminished, it is impossible to ignore the fact that many of the contemporary issues facing female doctors – raised within the subsequent chapters of this book – are echoes of themes presented in this chapter, fainter and weaker, perhaps, but still present. Women physicians, for the majority of their existence in Canada, could not easily be both a woman and a doctor. This was the result of both actual structural barriers, such as quotas on training programs, and the social and medical ideals that informed such policies.

Medical science has provided "evidence" for the inferiority of the female body since its inception; Galen argued that women were lesser, failed versions of men who lacked the internal fire needed to develop male genitalia (Laqueur, 1990). Indeed, medical historians and theorists have used this continued characterization of the female body as weaker and more prone to illness than the male to demonstrate how medical science reflected, promoted, and even created social norms (Ehrenreich & English, 2011; Feldburg et al., 2003; Mitchinson, 1991; Schiebinger, 1993; Warsh, 2010).

During the Victorian age, a crucial time of development for the medical profession, the primary governing social ideal was the doctrine of separate spheres – the idea that men and women were, by their natures, fitted to different tasks that complemented each other but did not overlap. Men were made for the public sphere, and women were deemed to be best at serving as "angels of the home" running the household, doing charity work in the community, and raising children within the private sphere of domestic life. Medical scientists, reasoning backwards from what they saw as self-evident social and Biblical truths, argued that only men's stronger physical body (as demonstrated by their larger size) and their clearly more developed faculties for reason (as demonstrated by both their larger brain size and the numerous historical successes of men compared with women in public life) fitted them to take on the challenges of the outside world including higher learning, business, and politics (Arnup et al., 1990; Bacchi, 1983; Carnes & Giffen, 1990; Mitchinson, 1991; Schiebinger, 1993; Smith-Rosenburg, 1985; Strong-Boag, 1979; Valverde, 2008).

In binary contrast to the idealized rational male, Victorian women were thought to be closer to humanity's natural side; as a woman's primary function was to bear and raise children, she was biologically ruled by her reproductive organs. Naturally capricious, these organs made women overly emotional. Their entire reproductive system was subject to the influence of the tides of the moon and any emotional shock could negatively affect the functioning of her uterus. Women's biology was her destiny; when controlled, her closeness to nature made her more intuitive, compassionate, nurturing, and morally inclined than men. Socially this control was provided by passing a woman directly from the care of her father to that of her husband. Increasingly throughout the Victorian era control was also maintained by regularly consulting another man: her medical doctor, whose job was to police her potentially wayward biology. As historian Wendy Mitchinson (1991) notes:

> The causes of ill health in women seemed endless – the way they ate, the way they dressed, their lack of exercise, marriage, celibacy, civilization itself. All conspired against them. Many were causes that could not be eliminated, for they were part of the social fabric of society… [and] women needed help, they no longer could assure their own health. (p. 14)

This gendered discourse of the Victorian era became a crucial and timely weapon in the medical profession's fight to consolidate and elevate itself. Since the beginning of the 1800s medical men throughout the United States, Britain, and Canada had been engaged in a project to redefine their profession as a learned, rather than laboured, occupation. As the days of "heroic medicine," so-called because of the extremity of the measures taken, waned, doctors wanted to be seen as gentlemen (Stanley, 2013). No more the barber-surgeon whose reputation was built on how fast he could amputate a limb in the absence of anaesthetics, prominent figures in the profession now made it clear that true medical men learned their craft in the institutions of the university and the training hospital – what is now referred to as the institutionalized biomedical model. More importantly, the claim of these new medical men to the right to practise through superior knowledge would be hitherto protected through legislation that forbade the practice of alternative, "quack" practitioners, including independent nurses and midwives, apothecaries, and blacksmiths with a "practis [*sic*]" on the side (Mitchinson, 1991). The worst of these would be banned outright and the others brought into the biomedical institutional model in a suitably subordinate position.

In this volatile professional environment, the gendered ideal of the angel in the home had profound value. The medical profession, which was almost without exception populated by males, were able to use the idea that women's bodies were naturally inferior to men's to convince half the population that their bodies, in particular their reproductive organs, were in constant need of medical attention; the medicalization of female reproductive processes, such as puberty, childbirth, and menopause, greatly increased their patient base. At the same time, they used the identical discourse to create a hierarchy within developing biomedical practice and to push out alternative medical practitioners. Only men, they argued, with their elevated capacity for reason could fully understand the scientific basis of the newly developed biomedicine. Indeed, any woman attempting to come to grips with such complex material would have to denature herself to such a degree as to place her reproductive organs in peril. "Success could be won only at the unacceptable cost of a coarsened sensibility" (Strong-Boag, 1979). The mental energy required would provide a dangerous shock to her system. Further, if too many women attempted this kind of brain work, the entire future of the race was threatened. Though this seems hyperbolic it was indeed a social concern for white, middle- and upper-class Victorian elites (Arnup et al., 1990; Bacchi, 1983; Smith-Rosenburg, 1985; Strong-Boag, 1979; Valverde, 2008).

These ideals not only discouraged women from entering an already overcrowded profession as doctors but also undermined competing independent nurses and midwives. During this time there were two classes of nurses. The newly professionalized nurses, trained in the institutional biomedical model to work as subordinate supports for male doctors, and their predecessors, variously trained nurses who worked independently of doctors and actually competed with them for patients. The discourse of the angel in the home supported only the former. Trained, subordinate nursing was viewed as a natural outgrowth of the domestic role, and the efforts of nursing reformers, such as Florence Nightingale, to make nursing into a respectable middle-class operation contributed to the development of the Victorian nurse as a hyper-feminine icon that was both sexually desirable and morally incorruptible – a perfect helpmate and binary opposite to the rational, scientifically trained, middle-class doctor that emerged triumphant from this period (Bates et al., 2005; Boutilier, 1994; Judd, 1998; McPherson, 1994; Stanley, 2013).

Some historians have painted this confluence of events as a calculated effort by medical men to continue and strengthen the historical subordination of women (Ehrenreich & English, 2011; Smith-Rosenburg, 1985). It would be more accurate to say that medical men during this time were able to take advantage of a social structure that benefited them, and by using that social structure, they increased its efficacy. Further, it would have been extremely difficult to counteract these social norms even if male doctors were inclined. Victorian modesty made it extremely difficult to conduct any examination on a living female, and in cases when a pelvic exam could not be avoided, young medical doctors were told to carefully avert their eyes from the form of the woman and proceed entirely by touch. It was also difficult to find any female cadavers for medical students to practice on. Even male bodies were difficult to obtain, and as fewer women died as indigents or criminals – the most acceptable sources for bodies – medical men had almost no training about the workings of the female corpus (Mitchinson, 1991; Porter, 1993; Richardson, 1987).

Given the hefty weight of such a social milieu, it should be unsurprising that most medical foremothers felt it was an impossible task to confront and deny the angel in the home outright. Indeed, given that Canada was especially conservative – more so than the United States and Great Britain – even feminists chose to work with the gendered image of women rather than against it. Unlike in the United States and Britain, where a majority of suffragettes argued for the female vote based on female equality, the deeply conservative first wavers in Canada argued for the vote based on their inherent difference from men. Positioning themselves as "Mothers of the Race," Canada's suffragettes argued that it was their inherent maternal and moral natures that fitted them for politics. In particular, they created their own powerful niche by setting themselves up as the protectors and spiritual mothers of Canada's poor, immigrant, and Indigenous populations whom they infantilized as needing superior guidance and supervision from women such as themselves. They portrayed this as both an extension of their natural mothering role and a modern extension of the charity work that elite women had always engaged in (Bacchi, 1983; Valverde, 2008).

This conservative feminist viewpoint helps to explain the directions of the gains made by Emily Howard Jennings Stowe, the first Canadian-born female physician to practise in Canada and the founder of the influential suffrage organization the Toronto Women's Literary Group. Stowe was born to Quaker parents in Upper Canada in 1831. As a Quaker, she was raised to believe that women were more equal with men than dominant society suggested and that education was the primary means to personal and social progression. The latter is of crucial importance as one of the main barriers to women entering medical studies was that they did not meet the required secondary school levels to pass the entrance exams, which required, among other standards, a knowledge of Latin. Many girls were automatically disqualified from even thinking about studying medicine because of the lack of secondary school opportunities for girls and women in what was still a developing nation (Hacker, 2001; Strong-Boag, 1979; Warsh, 2010). Stowe, despite having the necessary entrance requirements, was refused her application to study medicine at the University of Toronto because she was a female; instead, she went to Normal school and became a teacher. She eventually married John Stowe and had three children. Later, however, her husband became very ill and was confined to a sanatorium; Stowe would later point to that experience as the defining moment that caused her to apply to medical school again. Instead of reapplying to any of the Canadian universities offering medical programs and risking a second rejection, she chose to go to the much more liberal United States, where pioneer American female physician Elizabeth Blackwell had broken much ground and where many colleges were open to women seeking medical education.[2] Stowe graduated from the New York Medical College for Women in 1867 (Bershiri, 1969; Furst, 1997; Hacker, 2001).

Stowe's struggles did not end there, however. To stem the tide of doctors (both male and female) coming to Canada from the United States to practise, an act of Parliament had been passed in 1869 requiring any doctors trained in the United States to take one section of medical training in a Canadian school and pass the matriculation exam to

2 Many Canadian-born doctors also chose to practise in the United States, which was open to female doctors at a much earlier date (Hacker, 2001).

be licensed to practise. This was particularly problematic for women as no Canadian universities would accept them. Both Stowe and her colleague Jennie Trout, also trained in the United States, were forced to practise without licenses and, on a few occasions, were fined for doing so (Hacker, 2001).

Eventually, in the 1870s, the University of Toronto allowed Stowe and Trout to sit the necessary classes and exams for licensing. However, though the administration agreed in principle to women taking classes, it was not an easy experience. Not only did the students heckle, taunt, and play tricks on the two women, but they also faced discrimination from the lecturers who felt it damaged their own scholarly reputation to have to teach women. At the end of the process Stowe refused to sit the oral matriculation exam, stating she would not subject herself to the hostility of the examiners. Stowe continued to practise without a license until 1880. Jennie Trout quietly took the exam with no reported issues and became the first licensed Canadian-born female doctor in Canada. She set up a thriving electrotherapeutics clinic and a free clinic for impoverished women (Hacker, 2001).[3]

Trout and Stowe both wanted to spare future generations of women the discrimination they had faced at the University of Toronto. Instead of arguing that women deserved equal opportunities by attending co-educational instruction, they focused on setting up separate institutions where women could be trained as women. They thus tapped into a small, though growing number, of Victorian Canadians who supported female physicians whom they assumed would be more nurturing and kind in their treatment than male doctors and less likely to frighten vulnerable patients, especially children. These groups also felt female physicians would improve women's health overall as they would be able to treat those whose modesty forbade their examination by a male doctor (Mitchinson, 1991; Strong-Boag, 1979).

Stowe and Trout originally combined their efforts to open a Women's College at the University of Toronto. However, when Stowe stalled the

---

3 Jennie Trout was devoted to the practice of medical electrotherapeutics, which she credited as saving her own health from a debilitating nervous disorder. Yet most women who trained in such niche and, it must be said, fringe therapies, such as electrotherapeutics and homeopathy, did so not because they believed in their efficacy but because it was easier to get into those schools, which had less competition and tended to be less likely to bar women. Jewish women and non-white women in particular often found these they only avenues open to them (Warsh, 2010).

process, calling for more female control of the administrative levels of the school, Trout took her idea to Queens in Kingston (as well as her sizeable bequest should Queens agree). Stowe was furious, and the day after Queens agreed to open a women's medical school, the University of Toronto also agreed to set up a separate women's school. This meant that the two colleges were vying for what was an admittedly very small number of applicants in a small geographic area. In 1895, the colleges amalgamated, with the Kingston campus being closed in favour of the more central Toronto location (Hacker, 2001).

Women now had a place to study within Canada, but most hospitals refused to let women doctors in to finish the practical part of their training. To resolve this impasse, Dr Anna McFee, another medical foremother, again chose to use the discourse of women as different to found the Women's Dispensary in Toronto in 1898, creating a symbiotic, if unequal relationship, between the female medical school graduates and the local population of poor women; the former provided free care to the latter in exchange for gaining the required experience. This continued until the Women's College closed in 1909 when the University of Toronto's programs went officially co-educational (Hacker, 2001).

Historians are divided on the impact of the Canadian experiment in gender segregated medical training and its eventual demise (Hacker, 2001; Strong-Boag, 1979; Warsh, 2010). Certainly the Women's College provided opportunities for women not only to study but also to teach, which was crucial. While there were increasing opportunities for women to become doctors, very few were able to gain academic positions. It is also true that when Canadian universities opened their doors to the co-education study of medicine, many women found themselves running a daily gauntlet of abuse from students and teachers. Yet separate education also opened up female doctors to accusations that their training was less rigorous than in the male colleges (Hacker, 2001; Strong-Boag, 1979; Warsh, 2010). Further, while the college closed, the Women's Dispensary remained and in 1911 was made into a full hospital, which retained a policy of hiring only women doctors until 1961. It provided a place for women to gain expertise as well as a way for female doctors to create important networks of support with women in their field (Warsh, 2010). However, the Women's College Hospital was also a double-edged sword as it reinforced the idea that women doctors should confine themselves to treating primarily women and children; the problem of the segregation of female physicians in certain specialties remains a problem to this day.

Even though women now had places to be trained within Canada (other universities would open co-educational facilities) and ways to get practical experience and licensing, many still faced a society that refused to recognize that women could work as legitimate and competent medical professionals. The existence of the few Canadian women doctors complicated the "normality" of women's confinement to an ideological and physical private sphere. Many of Canada's first female physicians therefore chose to redefine their practise of medicine as falling within that private realm by reframing their work as a "mission," more as a holy work for God than for personal interest or gain. In the same way that suffragettes such as Stowe had redefined their activism to fit within the social structures of the day, female missionary doctors were able to argue that their natural female piety and compassion had resulted in their being called by God to serve, thus bringing public practice into the private sphere. Indeed, the missions provided both a bastion of encouragement for women doctors and potential places of employment.

As the Victorian and Edwardian eras came to a close, the British Empire, of which Canada was a part, was at its largest, and the Protestant and Catholic faiths were engaged in a spiritual arms race to convert these new populations as quickly as possible. Yet the Protestant missionaries felt they were at a distinct disadvantage by not having the same numbers of trained vocational people as the Catholic Church whose own missionaries, especially the various orders of nuns, had long histories of providing excellent medical, as well as spiritual, care. Thus, the Protestant churches, knowing that offering medical care was one of the best ways to successfully convert a population, became female doctors' staunch allies in the hopes they would spend at least part of their practice in God's service (Hacker, 2001; Strong-Boag, 1979).

Working as missionary-doctors, whether abroad or in Canada's largely unsettled west, gave female physicians an ideological way to reframe their gender deviance as compliance and, more importantly, removed them physically from many of the everyday encounters with a gendered hierarchy they would have to face working in Central Canada. Female medical missionaries reaped professional benefits while they espoused, and likely some believed, they were serving a higher calling. Historian Veronica Strong-Boag (1979) writes, "At a less altruistic level they no doubt appreciated the fact that in foreign fields they were afforded a level of power and authority they could never have at home" (p. 123).

Indeed, while the Victorian patriarchal culture disenfranchised female doctors at home, missionary-doctors could, and did, use aspects of the same social hierarchy to assert their power as upper- or middle-class white women over the local, non-white populations. Further, even if they went into missionary work with the noblest intentions, Canadian female doctors often displaced that culture's own traditional female healers, denouncing them as superstitious, dirty, and unfit to practice.[4] Those missionaries who were able to learn the language and understand and make allowances for differences in culture tended to be the most successful in the end. Dr Elizabeth Beatty was reportedly one of these women. Upon her arrival in India, rather than living with the large British-born white population in the area, she moved into a mud house among the local Indians both healing them and training them. The hospitals she established before ill health made her return to Canada were some of the most successful missions established overseas (Hacker, 2001).

Most of the women doctors who went overseas were single. Missionary life was often dangerous and incompatible with family life, and in the absence of reliable birth control young married female doctors were likely concerned about the issue of having a child in a remote and potentially dangerous location. For example, Dr Susanna Carson Rijnhart's husband was murdered by bandits while they travelled in Tibet soon after their infant son died of unknown causes, and many missionaries were slaughtered during China's Boxer Uprising in 1900 and the Revolution in 1911. Though India was safer in terms of local violence, missionaries regularly had to return home because of diseases such as malaria (Hacker, 2001). Further, if a missionary woman married another missionary, the church no longer viewed her as an employee and stopped paying her. Even if she was the only physician in the area, the church viewed her as fulfilling her wifely duty as helpmate and therefore not in need of compensation (Hacker, 2001).

Married female doctors often chose to become missionaries within Canada where their mission work could be combined with homesteading for income. Whether ministering to the few settlers in the new territories or attempting to convert the Indigenous populations, women doctors in the west were given many more opportunities to create a

4 In rare cases, however, these women worked together across cultures, often pushed to do so by the sheer lack of services where they were (Burnett, 2010; Hacker, 2001).

varied and challenging practice. Dr Charlotte Ross, a homesteader in Whitemouth, Manitoba, in 1881 actually never intended to treat anyone other than members of her own family. The other inhabitants of the area – mainly Indigenous persons and rough white settlers – likewise had little desire to be treated by a woman. However, in an emergency an injured lumberman came to their house looking for Ross's husband, hoping to borrow some first aid supplies. Ross cured the man but her reputation was sealed sometime later when she saved the life of a drunk man whose neck had been slashed open during a bar brawl. Unlike many of her contemporaries in central Canada, Ross was able to develop a highly unusual practice that did not focus primarily on treating women and children. Her patients were overwhelmingly male and, given the harshness of a frontier life based on homesteading and lumbering, Ross treated a large number of emergency surgical cases. Interestingly, Ross also used the harshness of her practice and her environment to highlight her own femininity. In the absence of other white women, Ross seemed ultra-feminine and the accounts of her patients – both male and female – remember details such as her consistently feminine dress and maternal manner (Hacker, 2001). The juxtaposition of Ross to both the environment and the other women, primarily Indigenous women, in the area meant she was able to claim the benefits of Victorian femininity despite her work.

Though being a frontier missionary doctor benefited a female doctor, it cannot be forgotten that the power they gained was often at the expense of the power of the local Indigenous populations. For example, Elizabeth Matheson trained as a doctor to help her husband run the mission in Onion Lake (in what is now Alberta), settling there in 1892. Matheson faced a similar bureaucratic issue as Stowe had in getting her licence. Having trained outside of the North-West Territories (as it was called then) she was not able to practise within it without taking the licensing exam in the same area. Because there were no medical schools in the North-West Territories, the University of Manitoba was designated as the exam site. Matheson refused because she had heard some of her male colleagues had been able to register without this requirement and because as the sole doctor in a remote location whose patients were primarily Indigenous, her registration was a largely moot point. Indeed, even though Matheson was not licensed to practise, she was still appointed as sanitary inspector in 1901 by the commissioner of health for the North-West Territories during an epidemic of smallpox. This meant that Matheson was in charge of enforcing the necessary quarantine measures over the local Cree people to prevent the spread of disease. After her success in that outbreak, the local Indian agent convinced the Department of Indian Affairs to appoint Matheson the official doctor to the Cree reserves; Matheson thereafter received a salary of three hundred dollars per year. Matheson did not bother to register for the majority of her career, eventually using her husband's influence to avoid the examination after several male doctor-settlers moved into the area and began competing with her for patients (Buck, 1974; Hacker, 2001).

Doctors such as Matheson represent the ambivalence of early medical missionaries practising in Canada's west. On the one hand, missions, such as the one run by her and her husband, offered much needed medical care to local populations. We cannot escape the irony, however, that the diseases that the Indigenous persons faced, such as smallpox, were brought by the explorers and settlers whose ultimate goal was to dispossess the Indigenous persons of their land and resources. Further, abysmal conditions on reserves exacerbated the experience of such illnesses, which increased the local people's reliance on the missions, which in turn furthered the mission's goal of assimilation of the Indigenous persons and the erasure of their ancestral culture (Burnett, 2010; Carter, 1990). Matheson's own story illustrates this ambivalence well. One of the main problems of all missions was erratic attendance by children at the mission school, but children were viewed as one of the main vehicles of successful conversion and assimilation. To combat truancy Matheson and her husband opened their home to many Indigenous and Metis children whom Matheson's memoirs, edited by her granddaughter, claim voluntarily boarded there. Matheson paints this situation as her becoming a surrogate mother to these young people, some of whom she would later adopt officially – a clear extension of the Victorian nurturing discourse. Indeed, Matheson is often portrayed as a mother to "hundreds" (Buck, 1974; Hacker, 2001). Yet the actual biological parents of these Indigenous children who lived at the Matheson mission are almost completely excised from her narrative. The story of Rosalie is one of the few that remains.

Rosalie was a Cree woman who bore a child to a white man who was not interested in Rosalie or the child, a girl she named Manias. Later, pregnant again and suffering from advanced tuberculosis, Rosalie asked Charlotte if she could place Manias in the Matheson's care. Matheson scolded Rosalie for getting pregnant so casually to a man she was not married to – clearly enforcing her own Victorian gendered and religious sensibility. Reportedly Rosalie replied that Matheson, as a white woman, could not understand what it was like to be "poor and helpless as we are to any man" (Buck, 1974, p. 68). Though it is impossible to know if Rosalie actually said this, Rosalie's story rings true to the experience of many women in her situation. Though Indigenous women could, and did, engage in voluntary sexual relationships with non-Indigenous men, as settlement continued and conditions for Indigenous persons declined, many Indigenous women engaged in casual prostitution to survive or were raped. Whatever Rosalie's situation, the missions often did not offer women such as her any real protection. Instead, all they did was take in their children, which served their own purposes of conversion and assimilation. In effect, Matheson colonized Rosalie's rights as a mother, and it cannot be denied that she used that colonization at least in part to build her own local reputation, which led to her appointment as a colonial official with a salary that helped her support her own family.

As the Victorian and Edwardian ages faded away into the horrors of World War I, medical science shifted, but the focus on female morality and the emphasis on motherhood changed little. Some female doctors did perform wartime service, though the majority were given temporary positions in Canada to release a male doctor to go to the front. Further, at the beginning of the war there was no way for women to serve overseas as they were barred from joining the military. Some enterprising and patriotic medical women did put together their own informal medical units and offered their service to the allies (Hacker, 2001; Warsh, 2010). These women made important inroads, demonstrating that women could handle the more masculine specialties, such as emergency surgery, as well as surviving the harsh conditions of war; these gains, however, were at best temporary measures accepted in the crisis of conflict, and most of these women's accomplishments were later dismissed as anomalous.

Unfortunately, the subsequent interwar period and Depression were not conducive to furthering women's issues and dominant gender norms remained firmly entrenched. Feminists are in part to blame for not changing the direction of gender discourse. Having won the federal vote in 1919 by basing their claim on maternalist ideals, those same women then applied the same discourse to achieving other social goals which usually centred on maternal, infant, and child welfare. In their bid to improve Canada and the people within it, they were aided by the increasing popularity of the "science" of eugenics (Gibbons, 2014).

Eugenics was attractive to Canadian feminists throughout the interwar period as it placed continued importance on the office of motherhood and served their own elitist agenda. Before and after World War I, leading Canadian feminists, especially those in the agrarian west, saw Canada as the country where civilization could reach its peak, being separate from the decadence of the mother country and ideological defiance of the United States. Social eugenics, the idea that parents passed on both biological tendencies and moral decay meant that the scourges of poverty, ignorance, alcoholism, and laziness all had to be stamped out so that Canada would not become a race of degenerates that failed to reach its full potential. If prominent feminists such as Emily Murphy and the Famous Five failed to "raise up" the population, each successive generation would be born more morally defunct than the last and Canada would fall. Several historians have noted how the eugenics and concomitant mental hygiene movements were ideal vehicles to increase elite Anglo-Saxon white women's control over non-white and working-class women: it gave them reasons to place the actions of those mothers under surveillance, and eventually that surveillance became formalized and codified into the emergent social work professions, aided in large part by the deprivations of the Great Depression (Dyck, 2013; Gibbons, 2014; McLaren, 1997; Samson, 2014). "This connection between progress, child rearing, and nation-building linked the individual and entire nation to maternity" (Gibbons, 2014, p. 130); by claiming that women were "mothers of the [human] race" and that elite white women were the supreme mothers of the supreme white race, these women put themselves in charge of anything to do with the family on a national scale (Valverde, 2008).

The idea that elite white women were supreme mothers of the race could even supersede actual biological motherhood. Women who had not had children of their own could still use this discourse to their benefit. Such was the case of Dr Helen MacMurchy. Remembered as one of Canada's first social reformers and more recently vilified for her support of the sterilization of the "unfit," MacMurchy was a trained physician, having earned her medical degree from the University of Toronto in 1901 at the age of 39. Despite the fact that MacMurchy never married or had children and reportedly detested the idea of a traditionally female domestic life, she used her role as a mother of the race to push Ontario authorities to examine the issue of infant mortality in the province. Politically savvy, MacMurchy called for the investigation with the clear idea that she would be its primary investigator, thus creating a job for herself. Afterwards she became the provincial inspector for the feebleminded, and in 1920 she was appointed to the newly created Federal Department of Health's new Child Welfare Division where she wrote the famous Blue Books designed to help mothers safeguard their own and their children's health in Canada's west (Dodd, 1994; Strong-Boag, 1979; Warsh, 2010).

MacMurchy was the first medical woman to be entrusted with such a high-level administrative position, which helped to crack a governmental glass ceiling, but she also serves as an extreme exemplar of the paths taken by many medical women during the interwar era. As the social administrative arms of medicine continued to grow, many female doctors were able to leverage the discourse of mothers of the race to become school inspectors and health inspectors and take up other local medicalized administrative positions (Dodd, 1994; Gibbons, 2014; Samson, 2014). Like the missionaries who used their position of power over local populations to turn the gendered discourse to their advantage, MacMurchy and her contemporaries turned the medical gaze on poor and often immigrant populations to create professional niches that fit the dominant gender norms of the day. As with the missionary-doctors of the Victorian era there can be no doubt that women such as MacMurchy believed that their actions were for the best; eugenics was the accepted medical paradigm at that time and would remain so until its association with Nazi Germany led to its discredit. However, their use of a social and medical hierarchy to empower themselves had consequences for other women, including the involuntary sterilization of women deemed "unfit" to reproduce throughout both Alberta and British Columbia (Dyck, 2013; Gibbons, 2014).

Throughout the first 50 years of women doctors in Canada, the majority of successful women physicians acquiesced to the dominant social-medical standards of the day. Women doctors worked within the social structures that limited them to nurturing roles and the private realm and, by doing so, made small changes and realized personal successes. In nearly all cases the women who were able to successfully pursue medicine during this time period were able to leverage power in other aspects of their lives, mainly their whiteness and class status, to overcome the barriers of their gender. However, even when the nurturing social female role could be successfully transformed via a godly mission or reformist impulse to create space for medical practice, that discourse also limited them and in many ways precluded the possibility of lasting change. Helen MacMurchy, for all her successes, was allowed to rise only so far; when the Child Welfare Division closed in 1934, she was forcibly retired and, because her sphere was limited to helping women and children, her skills were not as easily transferable to another department (Dodd, 1994). In other cases, it was women's own biological maternity that constrained them. In the era before reliable and easy-to use-methods of birth control, many of the Famous Firsts found their careers disrupted by maternity that could not be planned. Some, such as Emily Stowe and her daughter Augusta, created powerful female medical dynasties while others had to delay training or practice in the face of childbearing and lack of childcare (Hacker, 2001; Warsh, 2010). Charlotte Ross's experience took on elements of a farce. She trained in Pennsylvania and each year during the school break she would return to Canada to visit her husband. She inevitably became pregnant from these encounters, forcing her to delay her studies from the time she began to show until after the birth of her child. The situation continued throughout her schooling and her fifth child was born three months after her graduation (Hacker, 2001). Similarly, Matheson wanted to return to finish her last year of schooling when her then youngest child was only six months old. It was deemed socially impossible that Matheson's husband would care for a child so young, so Matheson placed her daughter with another settler who was by all accounts relatively unknown to her. When Matheson returned a year later to pick up the child, the woman was reluctant to let her go and the girl was understandably frightened to be taken away by someone whom she viewed as a stranger. Though Matheson's memoirs gloss over this account, it is clear the relationship between mother and daughter was never fully repaired (Buck, 1974).

Some women, such as MacMurchy, chose to remain single to pursue a career that remained at odds with at least the first years of child-rearing. However, even that was not a foolproof strategy as women were the traditional caretakers of their extended family as well. Well-known Canadian academic medical doctor Maude Abbott, the first female allowed to join Montreal Medico-Chirurgical Society, never married but her career was shaped by the fact she had to care and provide for her mentally ill sister Alice. Like many professional women today, Abbott relied on the help of paid caregivers to care for Alice and their household but, as historian Barbara Brookes notes, Abbott was still required to oversee all the domestic arrangements – a dual burden that saw her, and other medical women at the time, carrying a double load: "Unlike male colleagues who had wives who kept their households running, Maude was responsible for running their home in

St Andrews," including entertaining and other non-medical professional duties that could elevate or doom a career (Brookes, 2011, p. 182).

Given the severe limitations of working within the traditional female roles, it is not surprising they were abandoned as soon as possible. World War II saw some significant advances for women doctors, including their acceptance into the Canadian Women's Army Corps as full officers with the same pay as their male counterparts (Hacker, 2001; Pierson, 1986). Though the postwar period saw a return to the ideals of domestic femininity supported by new medical ideas of the female nature based on psychoanalysis, it seems few medical women tried to shift that feminine discourse to their advantage (Gorham, 1994; Mitchinson, 1991; Stanley, 2013). In postwar Canada, female doctors – sometimes called the second generation – dealt with their structural disadvantages in very different ways. No longer able to rely on women's and minorities' general lack of educational opportunities or science that "demonstrated" their inability to comprehend medical science, most Canadian universities enacted secret quotas limiting their enrolment (Duffin & Stuart, 2012; Hacker, 2001; Warsh, 2010). As historian and physician Jaclyn Duffin discovered, the University of Toronto's acceptance committee would go through each application accepting or rejecting it until the department secretary would inform them that the quota had been reached and no more of "them" would be allowed in; "them" referring to female and Jewish students (Duffin & Stuart, 2012).

Those women who passed through the quotas chose not to challenge the fact that they were never allowed to make up more than 10% of the class and instead, according to historian Cheryl Krasnick Warsh (2010), the second generation "left the feminist networks behind them and adopted wholeheartedly the male, objective, scientifically driven ideology of modern medicine" (p. 176). These women chose to live as doctors first and women second. Often married to male physicians who felt the same way, these women were aided by the advent of birth control, which helped control their fertility and allow them to conform more easily, at least, to their studies and practice (Gorham, 1994; Warsh, 2010). Indeed, some noted the flexibility of family practice, which allowed them to set their own hours and gave them more freedom than their counterparts in nursing who often had to work set shifts (Duffin & Stuart, 2012). They were also aided by the fact that medical students at the time were not required to have a degree before entering medical school, and a direct entry student could be practising as a physician at the age of 23 with plenty of time remaining to bear children if desired.

Now that the requirements have changed, many female physicians are forced to choose whether to interrupt their studies or early practice should they want to have a family (Duffin & Stuart, 2012).

Though many female practitioners found adopting a male physician persona was one way to circumnavigate the gender politics of their time, it was at best a partial solution. It often placed female doctors at odds with nursing staff who may have been their allies against workplace sexism (Gorham, 1994). In some ways the hidden, diffuse sexism of the postwar era was harder to confront than the overt discrimination of the previous era. Occasional ribald jokes or pictures in a lecture, the lack of appropriate female quarters for on-call doctors, and networking and team building events that took place in men-only spaces were ephemeral and thus hard to counteract. Second-generation doctors also were constantly having to disprove, in their everyday actions, the myth that training women doctors was a waste of resources since they dropped out to get married and have families anyways (Duffin, 2002; Duffin & Stuart, 2012; Gorham, 1994; Warsh, 2010).

Indeed, it would take the social revolutions of the 1970s to really start to make women doctors more than an interesting anomaly in the profession. The second-wave feminist movement, along with the patients' rights movements, civil rights actions, and the Red Power movement in Canada, exposed all the different ways that medicine had aided in the social control of non-dominant bodies. Having a female reproductive system no longer meant that a woman was doomed to periodic ill health and mental irrationality, and the right of women to pursue a career over having a family was finally recognized. But the echoes of the problems that plagued the first and second generation still remain as the rest of the works in this book attest. Family and medical practice remain an uncomfortable balancing act and one that disproportionately falls on the shoulders of women rather than men. If the past has two lessons to teach the next generation about how to deal with these issues it is that, first, women doctors must be careful not to obtain their power at the expense of other groups – a strategy even more untenable and unlikely to succeed in an increasingly diverse discipline and practice. Second, to create real change, we must challenge the entire social structure in which we live. Finding loopholes within a structure of disenfranchisement will only be at best a temporary and individualized solution. Women doctors must find solutions that allow them to be both women and physicians, rather than constantly having to emphasize one aspect of their identity over the other.

REFERENCES

Arnup, K., Lévesque, A., & Pierson, R.R. (Eds.). (1990). *Delivering motherhood: Maternal ideologies and practices in the nineteenth and twentieth centuries*. New York: Routledge.

Bacchi, C.L. (1983). *Liberation deferred? The ideas of the English-Canadian suffragists, 1877–1918*. Toronto: University of Toronto Press.

Bates, C., Dodd, D., & Rousseau, N. (2005). *On all frontiers: Four centuries of Canadian nursing*. Ottawa: University of Ottawa Press.

Bershiri, P.H. (1969). *The woman doctor: Her career in modern medicine*. New York: Cowles.

Bourgeault, I., Benoit, C., & Davis-Floyd, R. (Eds.) (2004). *Reconceiving Midwifery*. Montreal: McGill-Queen's University Press.

Boutilier, B. (1994). Heroines or helpers? The National Council of Women, nursing, and "women's work" in late Victorian Canada. In D. Dodd & D. Gorham (Eds.), *Caring and curing: Historical perspectives on women and healing in Canada* (pp. 17–47). Ottawa: University of Ottawa Press.

Brookes, B. (2011). An illness in the family: Dr Maude Abbott and her sister, Alice Abbott. *Canadian Bulletin of Medical History, 28*(1), 171–90. https://doi.org/10.3138/cbmh.28.1.171 Medline:21595367

Buck, R.M. (1974). *The doctor rode side-saddle*. Toronto: McClelland & Stewart Ltd.

Burnett, K. (2010). *Taking medicine: Women's healing work and colonial contact in Southern Alberta, 1880–1930*. Vancouver: University of British Columbia Press.

Carter, S. (1990). *Lost harvests: Prairie Indian reserve farmers and government policy*. Montreal: McGill-Queen's University Press.

Carnes, M.C., & Giffen, C. (Eds.). (1990). *Meanings for manhood: Constructions of masculinity in Victorian America*. Chicago: University of Chicago Press.

Dodd, D. (1994). Helen MacMurchy, popular midwifery and maternity services for Canadian pioneer women. In D. Dodd & D. Gorham (Eds.), *Caring and curing: Historical perspectives on women and healing in Canada* (pp. 136–61). Ottawa: University of Ottawa Press. https://doi.org/10.26530/OAPEN_578785

Duffin, J., & Stuart, M. (2012). Feminization of Canadian medicine: voices from the second wave. *Canadian Bulletin of Medical History, 29*(1), 83–100. https://doi.org/10.3138/cbmh.29.1.83 Medline:22849252

Duffin, J. (2002). The quota: "An equally serious problem" for us all. *Canadian Bulletin of Medical History, 19*(2), 327–49. https://doi.org/10.3138/cbmh.19.2.327

Duffin, J. (2010). *History of Medicine: A Scandalously Short Introduction* (2nd ed.) Toronto: University of Toronto Press.

Dyck, E. (2013). *Facing eugenics: Reproduction, sterilization, and the politics of choice*. Toronto: University of Toronto Press.

Ehrenreich, B., & English, D. (2011). *Complaints and disorders: The sexual politics of sickness*. New York: Feminist Press.

Feldburg, G., Ladd-Taylor, M., Li, A., & McPherson, K. (Eds.). (2003). *Women, health and nation: Canada and the United States since 1945*. Montreal: McGill-Queen's University Press.

Furst, L.R. (Ed.). (1997). *Women healers and physicians: Climbing a long hill.* Lexington: University Press of Kentucky.

Gibbons, S. (2014). "Our power to remodel civilization": The development of eugenic feminism in Alberta, 1909–1921. *Canadian Bulletin of Medical History, 31*(1), 123–42. https://doi.org/10.3138/cbmh.31.1.123 Medline:24909021

Gorham, D. (1994). "No longer an invisible minority": Women physicians and medical practice in late twentieth-century North America. In D. Dodd & D. Gorham (Eds.) *Caring and curing: Historical perspectives on women and healing in Canada* (pp. 183–211). Ottawa: University of Ottawa Press.

Hacker, C. (2001). *The indomitable lady doctors*. Halifax: Formac Publishing Company Limited.

Judd, C. (1998). *Bedside seductions: Nursing and the Victorian imagination, 1830–1880*. New York: St. Martin's Press.

Langford, N. (1995). Childbirth on the Canadian Prairies, 1880–1930. *Journal of Historical Sociology 8(3)*, 278–302. https://doi.org/10.1111/j.1467-6443.1995.tb00090.x

Laqueur, T.W. (1990). *Making sex: Body and gender from the Greeks to Freud.* London: Harvard University Press.

Library and Archives Canada. (2015, Sep 25). The Call to Duty: Canada's Nursing Sisters. Retrieved from http://www.bac-lac.gc.ca/eng/discover/military-heritage/first-world-war/canada-nursing-sisters/Pages/canada-nursing-sisters.aspx

McCracken, K. (2015, Jan 12). A Patchwork of Care: Midwifery in Canada. ActiveHistory.ca. Retrieved from http://activehistory.ca/2015/01/a-patchwork-of-care-midwifery-in-Canada/

McLaren, A. (1997). *Our own master race: Eugenics in Canada, 1885–1945.* Oxford: Oxford University Press.

McPherson, K. (1994). *Bedside matters: The transformation of Canadian nursing, 1900–1990*. Oxford: Oxford University Press.

Mitchinson, W. (1991). *The nature of their bodies: Women and their doctors in Victorian Canada*. Toronto: University of Toronto Press. https://doi.org/10.3138/9781442681811

Moscucci, O. (1990). *The science of woman: gynecology and gender in England, 1800–1929*. Cambridge: Cambridge University Press.

Pierson, R.R. (1986). *"They're still women after all": The Second World War and Canadian womanhood*. Toronto: McClelland & Stewart Ltd.

Porter, R. (1993). The rise of the physical examination. In W.F. Bynum & R. Porter (Eds.), *Medicine and the five senses* (pp. 179–97). Cambridge: Cambridge University Press.

Richardson, R. (1987). *Death, dissection and the destitute* (2nd ed.). Chicago: University of Chicago Press.

Rollings-Magnusson, S. (2008). Flax Seed, Goose Grease, and Gun Powder: Medical Practices by Homesteaders in Saskatchewan (1882–1914). *Journal of Family History 33(4)*, 388–410. https://doi.org/10.1177/0363199008323358

Samson, A. (2014). Eugenics in the community: gendered professions and eugenic sterilization in Alberta, 1928–1972. *Canadian Bulletin of Medical History, 31*(1), 143–63. https://doi.org/10.3138/cbmh.31.1.143 Medline:24909022

Schiebinger, L. (1993). *Nature's body: Gender in the making of modern science*. Boston: Beacon Press.

Smith-Rosenburg, C. (1985). *Disorderly conduct: Visions of gender in Victorian America*. New York: Alfred A. Knopf.

Stanley, H. (2013). Embodying family values: imaginary bodies, the *Canadian Medical Association Journal* and heterosexuality in Western Canada. In A. Perry, E.W. Jones, & L. Morton (Eds.), *Place and replace: Essays on western Canada* (pp. 207–26). Winnipeg: University of Manitoba Press.

Strong-Boag, V. (1979). Canada's women doctors: Feminism constrained. In L. Keeley (Ed.), *A not unreasonable claim: women and reform in Canada, 1880–1920s* (pp. 109–29). Toronto: The Women's Press.

Strong-Boag, V. (1991). Making a Difference: The History of Canada's Nurses. *Canadian Bulletin of the History of Medicine 8(2)*, 231–48. https://doi.org/10.3138/cbmh.8.2.231

Warsh, C.K. (2010). *Prescribed norms: Women and health in Canada and the United States since 1800*. Toronto: University of Toronto Press.

Valverde, M. (2008). *The age of light, soap, and water: Moral reform in English Canada, 1885–1925*. Toronto: University of Toronto Press.

Professionalization in Canada – An Annotated Timeline

HEATHER STANLEY

Introduction – A Historical Note

Creating a timeline of medical professionalization in Canada is somewhat akin to putting together a jigsaw puzzle that has no edges: there is some cohesion, but the boundaries remain ambiguous. This is due to several factors, the first of which is the sheer geographical size of our nation, which ensures that periodization of medical history is never exact. At the same time residents in Montreal were enjoying a multitude of medical services, including trained and licensed doctors, new hospitals and various public health schemes, settlers in the Prairie regions were making do without almost any professional medical care at all. Even now, the fact that Canadian provinces and territories, rather than the federal government, are largely in charge of delivering health care has led to regional differences in legislated medical practice, including who is able to practise medicine and with what title. Even today, only nine of the provinces and territories have reinstituted licensed midwifery programs and the provinces that have done so have taken different routes. Newfoundland and Labrador, though the youngest Canadian province (joining confederation in 1949), is also one of the oldest English colonies, which has given its medical history a unique flavour of new and old. Finally, fragmentation is exacerbated by the uneven study of medical history within Canada. Ontario's and Quebec's medical histories are the most well-documented, full of the details of medical discovery, and the founding of key hospitals and medical training facilities, while the Prairies, despite being the birthplace of medicare, remain largely uncharted territory, especially in the early periods.

Yet Canada's medical history timeline has many unifying features, including some that it shares with international medical histories, especially with the United States and Britain. Medical care has gradually moved away from a more diverse marketplace construction to a professionalized model, which reached the apex of social confidence between World War II and the social movements of the 1970s. The story is also one of competing interests: physicians, surgeons, midwives, and nurses sought to carve out professional territory for themselves and, in doing so, usually used dominant social norms and other social factors to bolster their own claims of expertise and authority. Though what follows is not intended to be a comprehensive assessment, it does provide some sense of the stages that different professional groups experienced as well as some of the effects of those movements on patient care.

Pre-European Settlement Era (1500–1600s)

In the pre-European settlement era, contact between Indigenous persons and European newcomers was infrequent or completely absent depending on a particular group's geographical location. Different Indigenous groups used a variety of medical remedies, and often caring and curing were tied to spiritual systems. Remedies varied depending on geography, with healers of both genders treating illness and injury with local natural resources and knowledges. When contact did occur between Indigenous and newcomer populations, diseases found new populations to colonize. Many Indigenous groups were devastated by illnesses of the Old World that their European carriers had developed some natural immunity to in previous generations, most notably smallpox. However, there has been some speculation that some sexually transmitted infections may have passed from Indigenous populations to the colonizers, notably syphilis. There is much further work to be done in uncovering the medical traditions and practices of different Indigenous groups during this time.

Exploration and European Settlement Eras (1600s–1850s, Longer in the Prairie Regions)

As Canada transitioned from a sojourner society to a colony, medicine remained, at best, rudimentary. Life in the fish and fur trade, along with agriculture, was harsh and accidents common. Much of the medical care was provided by women, and Catholic colonies had a distinct advantage because of the various female religious orders that deemed it their sacred duty to treat both settler and Indigenous populations; however, treating the latter was also part of their colonization and Christianization campaign and was highly raced. While some Indigenous persons were likely grateful to be treated, especially in the case of Old World origin diseases against which they had few natural defenses or local remedies, others were forced to abandon key elements of their culture to receive care. Indigenous persons also shared important New World medical knowledge with settlers – the cure to scurvy via boiling pine needles is the most popularized instance – often via intermarriages made between Native women and fur trader men.

The historical record shows that New France fared much better medically than the English Protestant colonies on the Atlantic coast, in large part because the services of the nursing sisters and the volumes of medical writing they brought with them. The majority of illnesses were still treated within the home, with home-based remedies often passed down orally or textually through the female generations, and usually combined with spiritual requests for intercession and cure. Even in cases where medical doctors were consulted, it was understood that any medical intervention worked only with the grace of God. Many women served as lay or fully trained midwives especially within the ethnic enclaves in what is now Ontario.

1600s Licences for medical doctors are distributed by regional authorities. Usually the only requirement is a degree from a recognized medical school in Europe. However, many practitioners do not bother to obtain a licence because of the high demand for any kind of medical services (licensed or not) in the New World.

1639 The medical mission that will eventually become the Hôtel Dieu is established by the Hospitalières order of nuns in Quebec. Other religious orders also provide various levels of nursing throughout the colonies.

1645 The Hôtel Dieu, thought to be the first major hospital in Canada, opens its doors. The nursing sisters who staffed the hospital are highly trained via apprenticeship in a variety of different vocations including midwifery and pharmacy. Some historians have argued that because cleanliness was part of the nun's spiritual devotions the hospital had remarkably low mortality rates for the time.

1700–1750s Quebec sets up a system of official midwives. By the middle of the century these women are paid by the state to serve the pregnant women of the colony. These women receive training at the Hôtel Dieu and also serve in the legal courts as medical witnesses. Unlike nursing sisters, these women see their work as midwives as a professional, rather than a spiritual, vocation.

1750 The Grey Nuns, also known as the Sisters of Charity, led by founder Marguerite d'Youville, open a General Hospital in Montreal that accepts patients of all classes. They also begin public health visits to the sick poor.

1755–1764 British-born and trained midwives are paid by the British government to serve colonists in Nova Scotia.

The Long Victorian Era and the Rush for Professionalization (1850s–1914)

The Victorian era, with the rise of the industrial city, was a crucial time for medical professionalization throughout the Western world. Previous medical training systems based on apprenticeship were being phased out, and institutional training and accreditation became important tools in demarking professional territory. However, medicine was still largely a private enterprise, as each transaction between a patient and a medical practitioner occurred on the basis of a business contract for services rendered. As cities grew new health challenges arose and the field of public health offered new opportunities for medical employment. Women, whose previous history of charitable work and "naturally nurturing" feminine temperament made them a "natural fit" for social work began to take many such positions especially in the wake of first-wave feminism. Social ideals about women's natural impulse to cure was also used by trained nurses and their supporters to advance their profession and aid its transformation from a form of domestic cleaning labour suitable for untrained working-class women to one supported by science, discipline, and cleanliness and therefore suitable for middle-class women.

1822 The first Canadian medical school, the Montreal Medical Institution (which will become McGill University in 1829), opens, but only for male students. This is a key development in medical licensing in Canada.

Before the opening of the first medical schools, a degree from any of the recognised medical training schools abroad or within the United States was sufficient to gain a licence from the regionally based licensing board. As more Canadian medical schools opened, they were able to exert greater control over incoming practitioners.

1850s Cities such as Montreal and Quebec City create local licensing systems for midwives. The Catholic Church follows suit in some rural areas in an effort to allow patients to differentiate between trained and untrained midwives. The Roman Catholic Church remains a staunch supporter of francophone midwives, who continue to serve both francophone and anglophone patients until the end of the century.

1850s The development of anaesthesia creates new treatment options, especially for surgery, and helps to increase confidence in physicians and surgeons. Surgeons are no longer evaluated on how fast they can perform an operation, but on how skilled they are in doing a procedure, which significantly elevates their status.

1854 Florence Nightingale begins nursing in the Scutari. Though her influence in the modernization of nursing has been debated, she would become a symbol of nursing as a trained middle-class profession for women.

1869 An act of Parliament passes requiring any doctor trained in the United States to submit to an exam at a local Canadian medical school. This makes it nearly impossible for women doctors to practise legally in Canada; though they could receive training at American schools that accepted women, they are barred from taking the examination in the Canadian schools. Later, when they were allowed to take the examinations many women would refuse to do so because they felt intimidated and were concerned about being failed because of discrimination.

1872–1881 Compulsory certification for midwives is introduced in Nova Scotia, New Brunswick, and Quebec.

1883 The Women's Medical College in Toronto and the Women's Medical College in Kingston are founded by competing Famous

Firsts, Dr Emily Stowe and Dr Jennie Trout. These all-female schools are founded in part to protect women medical students from the constant teasing and taunting that Stowe and Trout had faced in co-educational medical schools. The two schools compete for a fairly small number of female medical students within an extremely close geographical area.

1895 The Women's Medical College in Toronto and the Women's Medical College in Kingston amalgamate, the Kingston campus closes, and many Kingston instructors lose their jobs.

1897 Lady Ishabel Aberdeen founds the Victorian Order of Nurses (VON). The program is called for out of concern for the health of Canadian women settlers. Driven by maternal feminism, Lady Aberdeen and the National Council of Women attempt to form a district nursing and midwifery program modelled after similar systems of district nursing in impoverished English areas; the original name of the program, the Victorian Order of Home Helpers, is designed to remove any potential taint of charity that might make women refuse services. They are particularly concerned about the lack of maternity care for settler women who are often forced to give birth on their own or with untrained help from neighbours or their husbands. Without healthy settler families, Canada's potential would never be realized, and VON rhetoric was heavily tied to mythical ideals of the prairies. There is a huge outcry against the program by both professional nurses and doctors who feel that such helpers will encroach on their professional boundaries and livelihoods. The program then chooses to employ fully trained nurses instead. However, the fact that many of the nurses oversee maternity cases left them in a legal and professional grey area as technically only doctors are supposed to engage in such services. The VONs, as well as Red Cross nurses, serve western areas until after World War II.

1898 The Toronto Dispensary, which later becomes the Women's College Hospital, opens. It provides free care to poor women and training for female doctors.

1900s Midwives become "alegal" rather than illegal. They fall into a grey area as there is no regulation of their practice (unlike in other countries, including Great Britain) and they are not accepted as part of any provincial health care system, but there is no specific law banning their practice. Throughout the twentieth century midwifery falls into decline for a number of complex factors. The rise of confidence in science and biomedicine from the Victorian era casts midwifery as an unskilled and unmodern practice. Hospitals shed their previous association with charity, and as more options for pain relief are discovered, many women choose to have their babies in hospitals. Historians suggest that because Canadian midwives were a diverse group of women of different nationalities, training styles, and experiences, and because they were scattered across the vast geography of the nation, they were severely hampered in their ability to organize and professionalize.

1906 The Medical Council of Canada is formed.

1906 The Women's Medical College in Toronto is closed as the University of Toronto's medical program becomes co-educational. This is a double-edged sword. On the one hand, female medical doctors are no longer subject to the accusation that their medical training was inferior to that received by men. On the other hand, female medical students once again have to endure sexism from their fellow students and their instructors. Furthermore, most of the female instructors at the Women's Medical College lose their jobs and strict caps are imposed on the number of female students allowed to enter.

1907 The Canadian Medical Association (CMA) is officially formed from many local and provincial professional groups. The CMA is a professional organization whose goals include furthering medical science and, more importantly, protecting the interests of physicians against alternative medical practitioners.

1908 The Canadian Army Nursing Corps is founded as part of the Reserve forces. Their numbers remain very small until World War I.

1908 The Canadian National Association of Trained Nurses is formed to protect the interests of trained nurses against other practitioners claiming the title.

1911 The Toronto Dispensary expands to become the Women's College Hospital. The College Hospital provides a crucial training ground for female doctors to gain experience. It continues its policy of only hiring female doctors until 1961.

1911 The Medical Council of Canada creates its licensing program making medical licences portable across provincial lines. The lack of medical schools in the western provinces is no longer a barrier to settler-doctors, which is particularly important for female doctors.

1911 The Canadian Medical Association begins publishing the *Canadian Medical Association Journal* (*CMAJ*). The *CMAJ* provides a national forum for the medical treatments and discoveries of Canadian doctors, as well as a place for Canadian medical doctors to create and re-create their professional identity.

The Wars and the Great Depression (1914–1946)

The upheaval caused by two World Wars and the intervening Great Depression both helped and hindered the process of medical professionalization. During World War I many female doctors performed unofficial service by releasing a male doctor to go to the front. However, female doctors could not serve officially because there were no places for women within the Canadian military, except for nurses. Some enterprising women formed their own medical teams and offered their services to various allied groups. Nurses, in contrast were deployed as part of the Canadian Army Nursing Corps, which was created in 1908. Nursing was highly romanticized in World War I. The women who served were portrayed as perfect specimens of Anglo-Canadian womanhood, being both patriotic and feminine in dress, comportment, and role. Stories of nurses comforting wounded and dying soldiers, enduring privations, and working in harsh conditions became popular in war propaganda. Further, the poor conditions of enlisting soldiers in World War I combined with the privations of the Great Depression planted the seeds of many medical and social welfare programs enjoyed today, though their inception also signalled the end of many alternative practitioners, especially midwives.

Canada was much more organized in entering World War II, and Canadian women doctors were able to serve as full members of the

Canadian Women's Army Corps (CWAC). Crucially, CWAC officers, which included medical doctors, were paid the same as male officers. World War II also spurred a great deal of reflection about the kind of society that Canada should be – what kind of nation would be good enough to honour the returning soldiers. This social idealism led to many social welfare programs that had been proposed or tested during the Depression becoming permanent entities in the postwar era.

1923 The Canadian Government publishes a supplement to Dr Helen MacMurchy's popular work the *Canadian Mother's Book*. This supplement is designed for women living in isolated rural areas and contains a set of instructions for the "untrained neighbour" who might be called upon to assist a woman in childbirth. Though the book assures these neighbours they will likely never have to deliver a baby without the aid of a doctor because one would surely arrive in time, there is a realization that doctor assisted births in isolated areas are exceptions rather than rules. In truth, the book is an attempt to provide women with some kind of medical advice and service without resorting to the employment of district midwives, which MacMurchy and many other doctors actively opposed.

1924 The Federation of Medical Women of Canada is formed. Unlike the Canadian Medical Association, this group does not initially lobby for the rights of women doctors and instead serves more of a networking function for medical women.

1931 Midwifery in Newfoundland is legalized and regulated. Because of governmental concerns about high infant and maternal mortality rates and the remoteness of many rural communities, the government pays rural midwives to treat women in a series of cottage hospitals. These are usually staffed by women trained in Britain. Local "Granny Midwives," or local lay midwives, also continue to practise into the 1950s.

1930–1940s The development of antibiotics ushers in the "age of medical miracles" as diseases and infections that had previously been largely untreatable become curable. Confidence in biomedicine is at the highest in Canada during this time.

1940s–1960s Medical student quotas in major medical schools that limit the enrolment of women (and minorities such as Jews) are an open secret in an effort to keep competition for white male doctors as low as possible.

1944 Tommy C. Douglas and the Cooperative Commonwealth Federation enact Canada's first hospital and medical insurance programs in Saskatchewan. Hospital insurance is rolled out for the entire province and full medical insurance is provided as a pilot study in the town of Swift Current. Many doctors refuse to participate in the pilot study because they feel it will hurt their profits and autonomy.

1949 Newfoundland joins Confederation and begins to amalgamate its medical system with the rest of the nation. However, midwives retain their legal status in this province into the 1970s.

1950s The *CMAJ* runs several articles rallying doctors against any universal healthcare plan that would place them under the centralized control of the provinces. They ultimately fail to secure a program that guaranteed their autonomy to set and collect fees.

1962 Saskatchewan extends the pilot program to the entire province, granting all people in that province extended medical and hospital coverage. Doctors go on strike for three days to protest the move.

A Return to the Medical Marketplace? (1968–Present)

The passing of medicare, universal health care legislation, changed people's perception of good health from a privilege to a right. Canadians began the transformation from health care users to health care consumers. The counterculture movements of the late 1960s and the 1970s changed much of Canada's social landscape, including shaking the seemingly unbreakable confidence that biomedicine and medical doctors had enjoyed throughout the postwar period. Second-wave feminists in particular pointed out ways that medicine legitimized women's subordinate gender position by treating women as inherently ill because of their reproductive systems and by controlling how and where they received care. Feminist and back-to-the-land groups reinvigorated the idea that many medical processes such as childbirth were natural and should be treated as such. Many of their perceptions of pre-biomedicine life were highly romanticized, but their actions destabilized medical authority and paved the way for alterative practitioners, such as midwives, to regain status.

Over the next 40 years medical practice became both pluralized and yet increasingly focused on integration and standardization. That is, today, patients, provided they live in a major centre and can afford the costs of services not covered by the government, can choose from a variety of practitioners, including a medical doctor, a chiropractor, a massage therapist, an acupuncturist, or a midwife, and it is likely their care will be reasonably integrated and coherent across the different platforms. This is true largely because alternative practitioners have been increasingly absorbed into the biomedical model of standardized education, legislation, and regulation. While some argue this process was and is necessary to ensure proper standards of care, others point out that bringing alternative practice into the institutional biomedical model makes it less likely for people from lower socio-economic backgrounds as well as persons of colour to become practitioners, despite the fact that some vocations such as midwifery have a long history of being work for diverse groups of women. To be recognized as part of the medical system, alternative practices have had to conform to its standards of evidence, testing, and efficacy, which shapes their practice in particular ways. There has also been a trend to deskill several sectors of medical care to pay reduced wages to key workers. Nursing has seen its practice divided into several categories, with the lowest paid being licensed practical nursing (also called registered practical nursing) in which minority groups, particularly immigrants, are disproportionally represented. Eldercare in particular has been devolved to poorly trained and poorly paid care workers. Physicians are also seeing a shift in their practice as women doctors have been joined by some male doctors in calling for structural reorganization of private and hospital practice to allow a work-life balance, especially for doctors with families.

1968 Medicare is created. Canada receives nation-wide extended medical and hospital coverage. Private-for-pay medical treatment is made illegal.

1970s Indigenous women in the North are no longer allowed to be treated by local lay midwives. Instead, they are airlifted to the nearest southern hospitals to deliver. This causes a great outcry that continues to the present as many Indigenous women in the North prefer to deliver their children near their families and with people who speak their language and understand their traditions. Several women deliberately circumvent being airlifted by lying about their conception dates or seeking little or no prenatal care to force an emergency delivery with a nurse in local medical clinics. Unfortunately, an unintended consequence of such strategies is that women receive less prenatal care in their efforts to secure a local birth.

1973 Bette Stephenson becomes the first elected female president of the Canadian Medical Association.

1974 The Canadian Nurses Association makes a statement supporting nurse-midwives and suggesting their adoption as part of Canada's care system. This ends what had been a historical rivalry between the two groups over professional territory.

1994 Midwifery is regulated and legalized in Ontario. Indigenous midwives are still able to practise without regulation so long as they use the title "Aboriginal midwife" and serve only members of the Indigenous community.

1998 Midwifery is regulated and legalized in British Columbia and Alberta.

1999 Midwifery is regulated and legalized in Quebec.

2000 Midwifery is regulated and legalized in Manitoba.

2005 Midwifery is regulated and legalized in the Northwest Territories.

2008 Midwifery is regulated and legalized in Saskatchewan.

2009 Midwifery is regulated and legalized in Nova Scotia.

2011 Midwifery is regulated and legalized in Nunavut.

2012 Midwifery is regulated and legalized in New Brunswick.

2013 As no midwives have been licensed, the New Brunswick licensing body is eliminated. This means it is impossible to legally practise midwifery in the province.

3 Cultural Barriers within Medicine

SETORME TSIKATA

This chapter discusses the current culture in medicine and why cultural barriers contribute to gender differences in academic ranking and other disparities across the discipline of medicine in general.

It begins with the definitions of culture and cultural barriers within medicine and explores the history that has led to current gender disparities in the context of academic and non-academic medicine, followed by discussion of the consequences of these existing barriers faced by women, such as disproportionality in leadership positions despite increasing numbers of female medical students and faculty, and the importance of identifying and addressing these barriers. The unique position and challenges of women in medicine from a gender perspective are examined by exploring the natural tendency of women to be nurturing and protective in the context of culture and the healing process. The inherent responsibility women have to safeguard the sacred privilege of being entrusted with patients' illness experience, as well as the effect of differing cultural perspectives on the role of women – which partly influence the status of women in medicine – will also be reviewed. In addition, there will be a discussion about the challenges women face trying to balance their nurturing role and advocacy role in an ambitious field to project their gentle but strong attributes, that is, playing the roles of mother, wife, healer, teacher, and leader and striving to excel at all five. A chapter of this book dedicated to work-life balance will delve into this aspect in more detail.

Subsequently, the chapter will discuss the unintentional and intentional processes that contribute to cultural barriers faced by women in medicine, such as the over-concentration on gender gap in achievement, especially in academic medicine; the overemphasis on barriers women face in academic medicine versus non-academic medicine; and the superiority culture of specialists versus generalists, all set against the backdrop of the complex divide between and within the genders.

Barriers faced by ethnically and racially diverse women in medicine lead to less attention and focus on the vital and informative aspect of their diversity, in both academic and non-academic medicine; this factor is crucial and is discussed in view of the changing structure of the physician workforce and increasing diversity of women physicians occurring through immigration.

Other barriers faced by physically challenged women in medicine, as well as barriers based on religion, sexual orientation, social class, and age are also examined. In addition, an in-depth overview of cultural barriers encountered by women in various medical disciplines in provision of patient-centred care is discussed in a separate chapter on the effect of gender on patient expectations and biases.

Practical solutions from the literature for overcoming some of the aforementioned barriers are reviewed, including self-reflection and self-critique, cultural humility versus cultural competency, and provision of multicultural training of physicians – from undergraduate level through residency to the faculty level. This chapter concludes by proposing broad approaches to harnessing the opportunities presented by the rich cultural diversity among Canadian women physicians.

Definitions of Culture and Cultural Barriers within Medicine

Over the years, culture has been viewed and defined in broad and specific terms, without one universally accepted definition. Most definitions in the literature incorporate Franz Boaz's definition: "Culture is a system of shared beliefs, values, customs, behaviors, and artifacts that the members of a society use to cope with their world and with one another, and that is transmitted from generation to generation through learning" (Bates & Plog, 1990, p. 7). Culture also refers to the learned, shared, and transmitted knowledge of the values, beliefs, and lifeways of a particular group that are generally transmitted intergenerationally and that influence thoughts, decisions, and actions in patterned or in certain ways, according to Leininger and McFarland (2002). Tylor (1871, p. 1), a British anthropologist, wrote:

> Culture or civilization ... is that complex whole which includes knowledge, belief, art, morals, law, custom, and any other capabilities and habits acquired by man as a member of society.

Margaret Mead, the famous American anthropologist, also wrote, "Culture means the whole complex of traditional behaviour which has been developed by the human race and is successfully learned by each generation. A culture is less precise. It can mean the forms of traditional behaviour which are characteristics of a given society, or of a group of societies, or of a certain race, or of a certain area, or of a certain period of time" (1937, p. 17).

Building on these definitions, the professional culture of medicine can be viewed as the language, thought processes, styles of communication, customs, and beliefs that often characterize the profession of medicine (Boutin-Foster et al., 2008). In view of this, cultural barriers within medicine may be interpreted in a number of ways: hindrances or impediments to progress in the context of various specialties within medicine on a group level or between individuals making up the discipline of medicine as a whole. They may also be interpreted in the context of differences based on gender, ethnicity, race, sexual orientation, religion, class, specialists versus generalists, and other attributes with divisions or differences. Therefore, when a person of a particular culture encounters the beliefs and resulting actions of another culture, there may be antagonisms that decrease productivity, produce mediocre achievements, and negatively affect the goals and aspirations of the groups or individuals involved. The resultant dynamic is often far from cohesive and progressive and is instead fragmented, causing dissatisfaction on the part of those who live with and experience the repercussions of these barriers or who feel discriminated against. The following is a review of some of the relevant literature in the context of cultural barriers faced by women in medicine.

Literature Review

The published literature on barriers facing women in medicine due to their gender and other attributes both in and out of academia is extensive. Some of these barriers stem from the existing culture in medicine that tends to favour the career progression of men over women in the same field. Scholarship points to the culture of the work environment as one of the critical factors affecting women faculty's experiences both in and outside work (Brown et al., 2003; Carr et al., 2000; Foster et al., 2000; Levinson et al., 1989; McGuire et al., 2004; Shollen et al., 2009).

The intake of female students into medical school has steadily increased in the latter part of the twentieth century although, paradoxically, women physicians are a growing minority. Women make up 49%

of graduates but only 35% of medical faculty and 4% of full professors. Despite the fact that men and women share similar leadership aspirations and are equally engaged in their work in academic medicine, medical schools have failed to create and sustain an environment where women feel fully accepted and supported to succeed (Brown et al., 2003). According to Jagsi et al. (2006) there is a "gender gap" in authorship of the medical literature, and female faculty neither advance as quickly nor are compensated as well as professionally similar male counterparts (Mead, 1937). Consistent with previous research, no gender differences were found for either perceived job demands or emotional labour (Boutin-Foster et al., 2008).

A study published by Taylor et al. (2009) on career progressions and destinations in the National Health Service (NHS) of the United Kingdom found no evidence that women have been directly disadvantaged in their career progression in the NHS. Despite the fact that a smaller proportion of women than men progressed to senior posts, and men progressed more quickly than women to these posts, the career trajectories of women who had always worked full time were very similar to those of men. Men and women who had worked part time had broadly similar trajectories, which were slower than those of full-time doctors. It seemed therefore intuitive that the slower progression of women, overall, was attributable to the greater proportion of women than men who worked part time. Women with and without children achieved senior status at approximately the same time, and the percentages of women with and without children who reached hospital consultant status were also similar. There was no evidence that having children disadvantaged the career progression of women who had always worked full time, either in the percentages who reached senior posts or in the speed with which they reached them.

However, in the study, important differences were noted between men and women and between full-time and part-time working women in their specialties. This may reflect the perceptions of women about specialties that are relatively easy, and those that may be not as easy, for women and for part-time doctors to work in (Levinson et al., 1989). The over-representation of women in general practice, and their under-representation in hospital practice, is wholly attributable to the high percentage of part-time working women in general practice. A similar trend is seen in psychiatry, although the authors noted it was not dependent on full- or part-time work (Levinson et al., 1989).

Another interesting finding was that women who had always worked full time were actually under-represented in general practice. On the other hand, women were substantially under-represented in surgery overall, whether they were full time or part time workers.

Analysing further these findings gives an impression that women not progressing as far and as fast as men may be a reflection of not having always worked full time rather than because of their sex. The findings suggest that women do not generally encounter direct discrimination; however, the possibility that indirect discrimination, such as lack of opportunities for part-time work, has influenced their choice of specialty cannot be ruled out (Levinson et al., 1989; Jolly et al., 2014). Motherhood and other caring responsibilities may entail switching from full-time to part-time work, which will inevitably prolong training (Levinson et al., 1989; Jolly et al., 2014). Furthermore, lengthy training periods pose a challenge to women who want to start having children. Moreover, the reproductive years for women coincide with the age when most male physicians are at the peak of their careers and achieving great professional success. This creates a natural inequality that most women never really dwell on but embrace as part of their biologic processes, akin to the inevitability of menopause.

In her book on the slow advancement of women, Valian (1999) gives a convincing explanation of women's slow progress in the professional world of business, law, medicine, and academia, in comparison to the rate of advancement by men. She also points out that women are not paid as well, occupy less-powerful positions, and are not as respected as their male counterparts of the same level or rank. She attempts to explain why, and argues that we all have unarticulated, often subconscious ideas about gender that affect both our behaviour and, perhaps even more importantly, our evaluations of one another (Valian, 1999). She gives the examples of the idea that men are logical while women are social or the idea men are competent while women are flaky, leading to men being overrated and women underrated by coworkers, bosses, and themselves. The resulting advantages and disadvantages may be small, but they accrue over time to create large gaps in advancement (Valian, 1999).

The literature suggests that women working in academic medicine are disadvantaged both directly and indirectly (Taylor et al., 2009, pp. 16–19). Female academic physicians who work part-time and desire higher levels of scholarship in research, teaching, and clinical practice have the added burden of working extra hours to achieve the higher ranking of their peers who work full time.

Jolly and colleagues (2014) reported the results of a survey of physicians who received National Institutes of Health K08 or K23 awards between 2006 and 2009 and had an active academic affiliation at the time of the survey. They found that among those with a strong commitment to academic medicine, there were marked gender differences in the time devoted to domestic activities among those with children. Men and women who were married or in a domestic partnership without children had more similar patterns of time allocation both at work and at home, suggesting that the differences relate to gender differences specifically in the performance of child care rather than other household tasks. After various characteristics were controlled for, including professional work hours and spousal employment status, married or partnered female physician-researchers with children reported spending 8.5 hours per week more on parenting or domestic activities than their male counterparts (Jolly et al., 2014).

Women in Medicine outside Academia

While reviewing the literature for this chapter, it became evident that there was more emphasis on barriers faced by women in academic medicine than by those not actively engaged in academic or scholarly pursuits. Women in non-academic medicine, usually practising in community health centres or private practices, face challenges similar to their academic colleagues. Depending on whether they are in solo or group practices, the dynamic between staff and physicians and their respective belief systems may influence the culture in their practices. The good thing about out of hospital and non-academic or non-teaching practices (community or private practice) is the fact that women physicians have more elbow room to negotiate terms and conditions for their positions. There is usually not as tough a competition to rise through the ranks to reach the top per se. Physicians in private practice may not have the rigorous research and teaching obligations or be interested in these aspects of medical culture, compared to their academic colleagues. That is not to say they do not do research or teach, but there are no mandatory requirements for them to engage in these activities to stay employed or excel in their practices. They ensure that their continuing medical education (CME) credits meet the annual requirements to maintain their certification and licence to practise medicine in their chosen discipline (Burwick et al., 2011; Garattini, et al., 2010).

Medical schools depend quite heavily on community physicians for training of medical students and residents (Vinson et al., 1997; Dobbie et al., 2005). Some community physicians are affiliated with their local universities on a part-time or contract basis. Interestingly, some of these physicians who practise in their communities, outside academic institutions, teach learners in their private practices, may have first-year medical students shadow them regularly, and therefore play a very important role in education of medical students and residents that cannot be overlooked (Vinson et al., 1997; Bowen & Irby, 2002). Their contribution to medical education is not recognized appropriately, and they deserve to be congratulated to the same extent that their colleagues at academic centres are. There are often calls for volunteers to accept learners into their practices, especially first-year medical students. Many of these students are so inspired when shadowing their preceptors that they choose their specialties based on those interactions with these community physicians (Nieman et al., 2004).

So while their colleagues fiercely pursue their research agenda, community physicians also pursue the causes they believe in, such as mentoring first-year medical students, inculcating clinical knowledge and skill, offering guidance to avoid mistakes, just like their academic colleagues do.

Women in non-academic medicine also have the opportunity to engage in leadership activities within their medical community associations or specialty associations and offer their skills (in leadership or in other capacities) to advance the goals of these organizations.

A lot of lobbying goes into having women elected to leadership roles in their medical associations. The perception that an association fully embraces women to their highest offices adds clout and legitimacy to medical organizations, so there has been a gradual shift towards engaging more women in leadership roles, although success has been very slow (British Medical Association, 2016).

Culture of Superiority: Specialists versus Generalists

The culture of superiority associated with specialization and sub-specialization compared to generalists in medicine promotes discrimination in both subtle and overt ways. Specialists are paid more than generalists and more clout appears to be associated with specialization (Cheng et al., 2012). For women in medicine, this superiority culture related to specialization is likely to further impact their perception about their individual ranking among their colleagues if they happen to be generalists in their disciplines, and more so if they are general practitioners or do not belong to any of the traditional specialist fields.

Biology and the Unique Position and Challenges of Women in Medicine

Apart from the intentional and unintentional processes discussed that have created a gender gap in medicine, women have to accept their unique biology with its inherent attributes. Women by virtue of their biology and physiology tend to be nurturing and protective (Eagly et al., 2003; Magrane et al., 2012). Across the majority of countries and cultures around the world, women are considered motherly, with the accompanying attributes of being loving, empathic, patient, long-suffering, kind-hearted, and all the other "soft" maternal qualities, while at the same time, they are expected to be strong enough to multitask in coordinating domestic and professional duties. So in a sense, women physicians in their vocation try to balance the nurturing and advocacy roles in the ambitious field of medicine by merging the gentle and strong attributes – playing the role of mother, wife, healer, teacher, and leader and striving to excel at all five. As healers, the softer attributes auger well for patient-centredness; as patients' and women's rights advocates, the fierce protective attributes from the proverbial maternal instincts emerge.

Those women on the frontlines of patient care have the responsibility to safeguard the sacred privilege of being entrusted with patients' illness experience and to stand with them in their journeys either to cure or palliation, and this is where the softer attributes benefit patients and their families. Increasingly, patients want their physicians to be more empathetic and understanding, and most women physicians naturally play that role without much effort as compared to men (Berg et al., 2015).

Women by virtue of their biology are endowed with the ability to breastfeed – and males are not – so those crucial first few months in an infant's life require that women be available to nurse their infants around the clock if they so choose. Men are not equipped this way biologically and usually opt to continue to work or pursue their careers while their wives or partners care for their infant children, with a few exceptions who choose to go on paternity leave (Gordon & Szram, 2013). This natural phenomenon affords male physicians lead time in their careers ahead of their female counterparts who decide to have children during their reproductive years.

Women physicians therefore choose either to scale back on their academic pursuits to start and raise a family or to focus on their careers while putting off having a family, electing to remain single, choosing not to have children, or finding a balance of both on terms that bring them a fairly happy medium. Unfortunately, most women have difficulty finding a good balance and therefore become over-stressed domestically or academically, leading to burnout (Leiter et al., 2009; Gautam, 2001).

Influence of Cultural Differences on the Role and Status of Women in Medicine

Cultural differences emanating from disparities in the individual backgrounds of physicians who belong to a department, specialty, or university becomes an important factor when considering the dynamics between physicians, students, and residents in the workplace. These may include differences in gender, religion, race, ethnicity, or socioeconomic status that ultimately impact the role and status of women and their subsequent performance (Westring et al., 2014). Women from cultural backgrounds where males and females are brought up without any gender preferences tend to aspire to reach their highest potentials. There is a similar outcome for most women who attended co-educational institutions. However, women from cultures that elevate males above females tend to struggle with the notion of being on a competitive footing with their male counterparts and often require encouragement to seek promotion or ask for higher pay. They tend to be content with their achievements professionally and socially and are more laid back when the issue of salaries or promotions arise. Many women in this category value their role of raising kids and other family and social obligations above all other responsibilities. They are fairly content with their role and will argue to safeguard this personal decision whether influenced by cultural norms or not and may find women who desire the same opportunities their male counterparts have to climb the professional ladder sometimes too aggressive or even too feminist.

Stereotyping and Discrimination against Women in Medicine

Overt and subtle stereotyping and resultant discrimination occurs within the current culture of medicine. In addition to the challenges of pursuing a medical career when raising a family, female doctors sometimes report encountering discrimination and barriers to their careers (Burgess & Borgida, 1999; Heilman, 2001; Yedidia & Bickel, 2001). Discrimination may be direct, such as when decisions are made that favour men rather than women, or indirect, such as when women perceive that a career pathway is too difficult for them to pursue because of a male-dominated work culture, sex stereotypes, difficult hours, or informal patronage that favours men (British Medical Association Equal Opportunities Committee, 2004). Gender stereotypes have both descriptive and prescriptive components. The descriptive component consists of beliefs about the inherent characteristics of men and women. Central to these beliefs is the idea that women are communal (i.e., nurturing, kind, sympathetic, sensitive, agreeable, warm, and caring) and that men are agentic (i.e., assertive, aggressive, ambitious, competitive, independent, and outspoken) (Eagly & Karau, 2002; Heilman, 2001). These descriptive and prescriptive components leave women in academic medicine susceptible to stereotype threat in two ways; first, the assumption that women's communal nature makes them unfit for traditionally male (i.e., agentic) roles suggests that they are less able to lead than their male counterparts (Eagly & Karau, 2002; Heilman, 2001). Second, agentic female leaders in male-dominated fields who appear ambitious and competitive face violating prescriptive gender stereotypes and being viewed as unlikable and interpersonally hostile (Burgess & Borgida, 1999; Yedidia & Bickel, 2001). Women in academic medicine may be openly rebuked and disapproved of for behaviours commonly employed by and accepted in their male counterparts (Yedidia & Bickel, 2001; Pololi & Jones, 2010). This may lead to women avoiding violating prescriptive gender stereotypes (e.g. avoiding behaviour that could be interpreted as bossy or immodest) and may thus spend precious mental resources on impression management to avoid the very real consequences of either confirming or violating female gender stereotypes (Yedidia & Bickel, 2001; Pololi & Jones, 2010; Burgess, et.al. 2012).

Studies have found that women, but not men, expect to be negatively stereotyped (Cohen & Swim, 1995) and have lower performance expectations (Sekaquaptewa & Thompson, 2003) when they are relatively isolated from their same-gender peers.

The occupational sex segregation throughout academic medicine provides continuous reinforcement of descriptive male and female gender stereotypes and multiple opportunities for gender stereotype

priming, in which gender stereotypes are activated in people's minds, thereby increasing the likelihood that women or men will be perceived in terms of those stereotypes (Banaji et al., 1993). This is one example of the unintentional processes leading to barriers faced by women in medicine. This type of stereotyping impairs performance, such as when women are given tasks for which the criteria for success are framed in stereotypically male terms (Bergeron et al., 2006; Kray et al., 2002). There is considerable evidence that attributes for successful performance in academic medicine, particularly at the higher levels of leadership, are consistent with male gender stereotypes rather than with female gender stereotypes (Eagly & Karau, 2002). The mental model of a typical leader remains tenaciously male, especially in traditionally male-dominated fields, such as academic medicine (Eagly & Karau, 2002). However, studies of actual leadership effectiveness find little to no difference in the effectiveness of male versus female leaders (Eagly et al. 2003), but many experimental studies confirm the assumption that men are more competent than women with identical credentials in high-authority positions (Rudman & Kilianski, 2000; Sczesny et al., 2006; Rosser, 2003). Schein et al. (1996) coined the phrase "think-manager-think-male" to describe the phenomenon.

Sadly, the combination of the aforementioned dynamics leads to intimidation and suppresses talent, knowledge, and skills for the sake of portraying and adhering to the expected gender role. This pattern of stereotyping is systemic, beginning right from medical school throughout residency to faculty level. The systemic stereotypical assumptions about female residents and physicians still exist and are evident even in the language used in assessments and recommendation or reference letters, as demonstrated in qualitative research studies done by Schmader et al. (2007) and Isaac (2011). The authors raise intriguing questions in these two papers including, "Why do women have to anticipate others' needs and 'get their confidence?" This type of language raises doubt (Schmader et al., 2007) about these women students' roles and abilities.

On one hand, male writers thought it important that women students accomplish tasks without being prompted and to recognize their deficits. On the other hand, female writers know the importance of independence for the physician trainees but stating "functions independently" blurs the word independence. This becomes counterproductive to progress and to women's academic development.

Stereotyping and Discrimination against International Medical Graduates – Interplay of Gender and Racial Biases

Another form of stereotyping which affects men and women equally in medicine is the notion that international medical graduates (IMGs) are less competent than their North American or western-trained counterparts in certain aspects of medical practice (Rojas et al., 2011). Research shows that foreign medical graduates who are largely first-generation immigrants face added prejudice and are discriminated against very or somewhat significantly (Coombs & King, 2005), either overtly or in subtle ways, based on chauvinistic attitudes, xenophobia, and their country of origin (Desbiens & Vidaillet, 2010). In Coombs et al.'s (2005) survey of 445 licensed physicians in Massachusetts, more than 60% of respondents reported that discrimination against foreign medical graduates was very or somewhat significant, while 44% of US medical graduates reported that discrimination against foreign medical graduates in their present organization was significant. Moreover, there are relatively fewer foreign medical graduates than American graduates in competitive, financially lucrative specialties (Brotherton & Etzel, 2010). Surgery in particular is infamous for discriminating against foreign medical graduates, with some surgical directors acknowledging external pressure to rank a US medical graduate over a better-qualified foreign medical graduate (Desbiens & Vidaillet, 2010).

The interplay of gender and racial discrimination is an interesting one in all disciplines, and medicine has had its share of experiences. For instance, Murti (2012) found that Indian male physicians enjoyed social acceptance on revealing their occupational status, whereas Indian female physicians were seen as more intimidating socially and risked social marginalization for seizing high social status reserved for white men. So, for minority women and generally women of colour in medicine, gender and racial discrimination become a double bind and lead to higher levels of discrimination (Carr et al., 2007). In the same vein, (Gray et al., 1996) report substantial differences in perceptions for women and minority graduates compared to white male graduates regarding experiences at medical school and the professional medical environment in the United States. Minority faculty members report lower levels of satisfaction (Palepu et al., 2000) and are more likely to leave their academic careers (Hadley et al., 1992).

This is a very complex and sensitive area of discussion and needs to be put in context when debating to what extent this stereotyping is real. There are disparities in the curricula of medical schools, between countries, continents, and individual institutions. Developing countries tend to focus more on infectious diseases than the west does, where more emphasis is placed on cardiovascular health, oncology, and preventive care among other areas. This may lead to subtle differences in management options on either side. Another crucial factor is how IMGs immigrated to western countries to practise. Every individual IMG has his or her own story of how they came to be practising medicine in the west. These reasons may span from displacement through wars, natural disasters, religious persecution, political dissentions, or simply for a better life or for the desire to relocate to pursue a better livelihood for their families. Whatever the reasons may be, they are usually required to write and pass exams and retrain in their field of expertise if they have been out of practice for more than a couple of years. Women IMGs tend to bear the bigger brunt of this stereotyping because of the longer time they may have been out of training or academia if they were raising a family, for instance or needed temporary employment to earn a living while waiting to get their license to practice. A typical example is the instance when both husband and wife are physicians, and they can only afford to have one person studying at a time. One male physician from South Asia said he decided his wife, who is also a physician, should stay home and raise their children while he pursues his certification to practise medicine in a North American country. This was a decision they were apparently both comfortable with. There are many such stories, including from those who have been displaced for many years and have lost most of their clinical knowledge and skills; they are unprepared to practise medicine without refresher courses or upgrading their clinical skills.

In view of these examples, painting IMGs with a broad brush as being incompetent or having substandard training is misplaced. After all, many IMGs have gone on to excel and do outstanding work both in the west and internationally and made an impact in medicine and science as a whole.

Visible minority women physicians also experience various forms of discrimination by virtue of differences in their race or ethnicity, especially in Caucasian dominated medical schools. Some report having to work twice as hard to gain half the recognition accorded to their male and female counterparts. Having only a small pool of mentors to look up too, these women face more hurdles than their Caucasian sisters when they need support to further their careers.

Speaking of sisterhood, some women physicians have issues with the handful of their colleagues who have made it to top positions in academia or other fields in medicine because they feel left behind. The hope is that when women get to the top, they will remember those left at the bottom and fight on their behalf. Some cynics term it the "female phenomenon" where a few women get to the pinnacle of their career and want to own that space while men usually welcome their friends from the "old boys club" to join them at the top. Whether this is a myth or is real remains to be seen. On the other hand, some women leaders have fiercely sought to keep trusted female colleagues on their teams and give opportunities to younger female colleagues through collaboration and mentorship in various aspects of their work (e.g., teaching, practice, and research).

Despite the entrenchment of gendered and racialized assumptions and expectations within the practices of these organizations, most research ignores how the gender category is deeply complicated by racial and ethnic differences (Acker, 2006). Focusing on any one category ignores the internal divisions of races along gender and nationality lines, and precludes an understanding of how these categories have a complex, mutually reinforcing or contradicting interaction (Bhatt, 2013).

Discrimination on the Basis of Religion, Sexual Orientation, and Physical and Neuropsychological Ability

Other discrimination faced by women hinges on their sexuality or religious affiliation. Physicians who are gay are often the target of gossip for their superiors, colleagues, students, and patients. Some patients may even decline to be attended to by a gay physician and colleagues may opt out of working on the same project with them if given the option. Women with religious beliefs that require them to take a submissive role both at home to their husbands and at work to other men may come across as overly passive and unengaging and lose out on opportunities for promotion or advancement in their careers. These women find it their sacred religious duty to defer decision making to their male counterparts, which may be seen by others as anti-feminist. It creates a false sense of a defeatist attitude when observed by those outside that particular religion. Women in this position have to deal with the internal conflict of the expectations of independence when this fundamentally violates their religious beliefs. There is a similar trend for women who choose not to attend to male patients for religious or cultural reasons. For those who are obligated to wear clothing that visibly identifies them as belonging to a particular religion (e.g., the hijab for Muslim women), the impact of such discrimination is more pronounced such that in anecdotal reports, they have been targeted by non-adherents.

Women who have physical disabilities may not be adequately physically accommodated. Those with disorders such as Tourette syndrome, bipolar affective disorder, or obsessive compulsive disorder may find it challenging working in the same environment with other physicians without the required psychological supports and accommodation to function effectively.

Consequences of Cultural Barriers Faced by Women in Medicine

As a result of the cultural barriers faced by women in medicine, there is disproportionality in leadership positions for women, despite the increasing number of female medical students, residents, and faculty. Female medical students advance through university watching more men climb the leadership ladder and their female counterparts remain somewhat stagnant at the same positions through residency until they enter independent practice in their chosen disciplines. Witnessing this trend likely leaves a subtle image of male dominance, which can unconsciously become acceptable to female students who then attain faculty membership and are content with the status quo. This is compounded by fewer female physician mentors/leaders compared to male physicians who can be role models to help young people see leadership roles as achievable equally by both men and women.

Unfortunately, as this trend continues, talent and skill in women remains untapped because of the fear of being labelled as being either too assertive or too abrasive if they occupy leadership positions or aspire to run for leadership positions in their departments or medical associations. This unconsciously perpetuates a pseudo-culture of mediocrity and ambivalence. On one hand, women in medicine want to do as well as their male counterparts, but on the other hand, most wonder whether it is worth fighting to break the barriers that currently exist, only to be met with the negative stereotyping discussed. Gender and racial discrimination thus act as a double bind for minority women in medicine, who, when compared to men, report higher levels of discrimination (Carr et al., 2007).

Inevitably, the same biases and stereotypical behaviour seen among women in academic medicine is also seen in non-academic settings. It speaks to a broader culture of gender bias and cannot be dichotomized based on academia alone.

Importance of Identifying and Addressing Cultural Barriers Women Face in Medicine

Without purposefully and consciously engaging in discussions about barriers women face in medicine, it is easy to ignore the problem, especially because of the spurious idea that since the intake of women into medical disciplines is increasing, women now have a level playing field with their male colleagues in both academic and non-academic achievements and progression or advancement in medicine as a whole. Without acknowledgment that barriers still exist, there will be no opportunity to work at finding solutions to break down these barriers and bridge the divide between male and female physicians' advancement in Medicine. This is why it is important to encourage an honest and open discussion about the status quo.

Women who already are on shaky ground because of their slow progress on the academic track may not be eager to identify and discuss some of the aforementioned challenges, more so if they are of visible minority group. Some value the rare opportunity of being among their majority counterparts and would rather choose the battles they fight carefully. Others recognize the culture of having visible minorities, especially females, to lend to the optics of fairness and equity and are content to play the part and not rock the boat. It is typically easier for the few women who are "privileged" enough to have their hard work and achievements recognized in leadership positions to trumpet the above concerns without reprisal from their male and female colleagues alike.

Proposed Solutions

In Valian's book (1999) on the slow advancement of women in medicine, the chapter on remedies offers specific ways to mitigate the negative professional consequences of gender schemas. She contends that the most common professional outcome of gender schemas is the under-evaluation of women's performance. But before we can change this structure formally, we must take a look at both others' and our own behaviour and become aware of the strong but not always obvious presence of gender schemas (Valian, 1999). It is also critical that physicians recognize the differences in the domestic activities of male and female physicians and specifically among those who are members of a generation in which gender equity is generally embraced. Such awareness is essential for the appropriate development of interventions to promote the success of both men and women (Taylor et al., 2009).

Concrete strategies from the literature to reduce the effects of stereotype threat for female faculty members at academic health centres include the following strategies discussed by Burgess et al. (2012):

- Introduce the concept of stereotype threat to the academic medicine community
- Engage all stakeholders, male and female, to promote identity safety
- Counteract the effects of occupational sex segregation at academic health centres
- Reduce gender stereotype priming
- Build leadership efficacy among female physicians and scientists

Organizations can improve women's ability to achieve their full potential by taking measures to nurture female talent (Nath et al., 2014). Support from male and female leaders can set the tone and direction for the whole organization. Strategies including mentoring, career planning, equity recruitment planning, and talent spotting all undoubtedly help and should be part of these efforts. The focus now should be on medical institutions to increase the representation of women in leadership positions by recognizing barriers and strategizing to overcome them. There must be committed senior leadership, giving clear messages of support and ensuring there are measurable systems and active mentoring programs in place to support women's careers (Nath et al., 2014).

Women in medicine holding leadership positions can volunteer their time and effort to mobilize junior female physicians and residents/students through networking, exchanging ideas, and counselling where needed. Supporting national women physician organizations, such as the Federation of Medical Women of Canada, a national branch of the international organization Medical Women International Association, mentorship groups that foster collaboration and promote the well-being and advancement of female physicians, will encourage women in medicine to strive to achieve greater heights.

Diversity among women in medicine should be embraced. IMGs should be encouraged to contribute their wealth of experience to help serve the increasingly diverse population that is emerging world-wide. Self-reflection and self-critique, cultural humility, cultural competency, and multicultural training of physicians from undergraduate level through residency to the faculty level are strategies that can help curb some of the stereotypical attitudes that currently exist towards IMGs and visible minority women in medicine.

Conclusion

Not all physicians can pursue purely academic medicine in view of the natural and artificial barriers, and those created through intentional and unintentional processes. No matter which category a female practising medicine falls into, she should be able to choose a path that fulfills her either in a traditional role of maintaining a career and earning a decent living without the pressures of stringent professional or academic expectations, to pursue advancement professionally and academically with all the available opportunities that male physicians have, or to combine the two. Ideally, there should be structures to support either of these choices by all institutions. But most importantly, the culture in medicine needs a fundamental paradigm shift to embrace the strengths and address the weaknesses of all genders, equally, irrespective of race, ethnicity, religion, physical and neuropsychological ability, or country of origin or training; to promote diversity and the advancement of all members of the medical community; and to correct the inequality that currently exists in the process.

REFERENCES

Bates, D.G., & Plog, F. (1990). *Cultural anthropology* (3rd ed.). New York: McGraw-Hill.

British Medical Association. (2016, Jun 30). Wanted: Women leaders. Retrieved from http:/www.bma.org.uk/news-views-analysis/news/2014/january/wanted-women-leaders

British Medical Association Equal Opportunities Committee. (2004). Career barriers in medicine: Doctors' experiences. Retrieved from http://*www.hscbusiness.hscni.net/pdf/BMA-_Career_Barriers_in_Medicine-2004_pdf.pdf*

Acker, J. (2006). Inequality regimes: Gender, class, and race in organizations. *Gender & Society, 20*(4), 441–64. https://doi.org/10.1177/0891243206289499

Banaji, M.R., Hardin, C., & Rothman, A.J. (1993). Implicit stereotyping in person judgment. *Journal of Personality and Social Psychology, 65*(2), 272–81. https://doi.org/10.1037/0022-3514.65.2.272

Berg, K., Blatt, B., Lopreiato, J., Jung, J., Schaeffer, A., Heil, D., …, & Hojat, M. (2015, Jan). Standardized patient assessment of medical student empathy: Ethnicity and gender effects in a multi-institutional study. *Academic Medicine: Journal of the Association of American Medical College, 90*(1), 105–11. https://doi.org/10.1097/ACM.0000000000000529 Medline:25558813

Bergeron, D.M., Block, C.J., & Echtenkamp, B.A. (2006). Disabling the able: Stereotype threat and women's work performance. *Human Performance, 19*(2), 133–58. https://doi.org/10.1207/s15327043hup1902_3

Bhatt, W. (2013). The little brown woman: Gender discrimination in American medicine. *Gender & Society, 27*(5), 659–80. https://doi.org/10.1177/0891243213491140

Boutin-Foster, C., Foster, J.C., & Konopasek, L. (2008, Jan). Viewpoint: Physician, know thyself: The professional culture of medicine as a framework for teaching cultural competence. *Academic Medicine: Journal of the Association of American Medical College, 83*(1), 106–11. https://doi.org/10.1097/ACM.0b013e31815c6753 Medline:18162762

Bowen, J.L., & Irby, D.M. (2002, Jul). Assessing quality and costs of education in the ambulatory setting: A review of the literature. *Academic Medicine: Journal of the Association of American Medical College, 77*(7), 621–80. https://doi.org/10.1097/00001888-200207000-00006 Medline:12114139

Brotherton, S.E., & Etzel, S.I. (2010). Graduate medical education, 2009–2010. *JAMA, 304*(11), 1255–70. https://doi.org/10.1001/jama.2010.1273 Medline:20841543

Brown, A.J., Swinyard, W., & Ogle, J. (2003, Dec). Women in academic medicine: A report of focus groups and questionnaires, with conjoint analysis. *Journal of Women's Health (2002), 12*(10), 999–1008. https://doi.org/10.1089/154099903322643929 Medline:14709188

Burgess, D., & Borgida, E. (1999). Who women are, who women should be – Descriptive and prescriptive gender stereotyping in sex discrimination. *Psychology, Public Policy, and Law, 5*(3), 665–92. https://doi.org/10.1037/1076-8971.5.3.665

Burgess, D.J., Joseph, A., van Ryn, M., & Carnes, M. (2012, Apr). Does stereotype threat affect women in academic medicine? *Academic Medicine: Journal of the Association of American Medical College, 87*(4), 506–12. https://doi.org/10.1097/ACM.0b013e318248f718 Medline:22361794

Burwick, R.M., Schulkin, J., Cooley, S.W., Janakiraman, V., Norwitz, E.R., & Robinson, J.N. (2011, May). Recent trends in continuing medical education among obstetrician-gynecologists. *Obstetrics and Gynecology, 117*(5), 1060–4. https://doi.org/10.1097/AOG.0b013e318214e561 Medline:21508743

Carr, P.L., Ash, A.S., Friedman, R.H., Szalacha, L., Barnett, R.C., Palepu, A., & Moskowitz, M.M. (2000). Faculty perceptions of gender discrimination and sexual harassment in academic medicine. *Annals of Internal Medicine, 132*(11), 889–96. https://doi.org/10.7326/0003-4819-132-11-200006060-00007 Medline:10836916

Carr, P.L., Palepu, A., Szalacha, L., Caswell, C., & Inui, T. (2007). "Flying below the radar": A qualitative study of minority experience and management of discrimination in academic medicine. *Medical Education, 41*(6), 601–9. https://doi.org/10.1111/j.1365-2923.2007.02771.x Medline:17518841

Cheng, T.C., Scott, A., Jeon, S.-H., Kalb, G., Humphreys, J., & Joyce, C. (2012, Nov). What factors influence the earnings of general practitioners and medical specialists? Evidence from the medicine in Australia: Balancing employment and life survey. *Health Economics, 21*(11), 1300–17. https://doi.org/10.1002/hec.1791 Medline:21919116

Cohen, L.L., & Swim, J.K. (1995). The differential impact of gender ratios on women and men: Tokenism, self-confidence, and expectations. *Personality and Social Psychology Bulletin, 21*(9), 876–84. https://doi.org/10.1177/0146167295219001

Coombs, A.A.T., & King, R.K. (2005). Workplace discrimination: Experiences of practicing physicians. *Journal of the National Medical Association, 97*(4), 467–77. Medline:15868767

Desbiens, N.A., & Vidaillet, H.J., Jr. (2010). Discrimination against international medical graduates in the United States residency program selection process. *BMC Medical Education, 10*(1), 5. https://doi.org/10.1186/1472-6920-10-5 Medline:20100347

Dobbie, A.E., Tysinger, J.W., & Freeman, J. (2005). Strategies for efficient office precepting. *Family Medicine, 37*(4), 239–41. Medline:15812687

Eagly, A.H., Johannesen-Schmidt, M.C., & van Engen, M.L. (2003). Transformational, transactional, and laissez-faire leadership styles: A meta-analysis comparing women and men. *Psychological Bulletin, 129*(4), 569–91. https://doi.org/10.1037/0033-2909.129.4.569 Medline:12848221

Eagly, A.H., & Karau, S.J. (2002). Role congruity theory of prejudice toward female leaders. *Psychological Review, 109*(3), 573–98. https://doi.org/10.1037/0033-295X.109.3.573 Medline:12088246

Foster, S.W., McMurray, J.E., Linzer, M., Leavitt, J.W., Rosenberg, M., & Carnes, M. (2000, Jun). Results of a gender-climate and work-environment survey at a midwestern academic health center. *Academic Medicine: Journal of the Association of American Medical College, 75*(6), 653–60. https://doi.org/10.1097/00001888-200006000-00019 Medline:10875512

Garattini, L., Gritti, S., De Compadri, P., & Casadei, G. (2010, Mar). Continuing medical education in six European countries: A comparative analysis. *Health Policy (Amsterdam, Netherlands)*, *94*(3), 246–54. https://doi.org/10.1016/j.healthpol.2009.09.017 Medline:19913324

Gautam, M. (2001, Jan). Women in medicine: Stresses and solutions. *The Western Journal of Medicine*, *174*(1), 37–41. https://doi.org/10.1136/ewjm.174.1.37 Medline:11154666

Gordon, H., & Szram, J. (2013, Oct). Paternity leave experiences of NHS doctors. *Clinical Medicine (London, England)*, *13*(5), 426–30. https://doi.org/10.7861/clinmedicine.13-5-426 Medline:24115693

Gray, G.M., Gallagher, T.C., & Masters, M.S. (1996). Contrasting experiences and perceptions of women and men physician graduates of Stanford University School of Medicine. *Transactions of the American Clinical and Climatological Association*, *107*, 159–74. Medline:8725569

Hadley, J., Cantor, J.C., Willke, R.J., Feder, J., & Cohen, A.B. (1992, Mar). Young physicians most and least likely to have second thoughts about a career in medicine. *Academic Medicine: Journal of the Association of American Medical Colleges*, *67*(3), 180–90. https://doi.org/10.1097/00001888-199203000-00010 Medline:1540272

Heilman, M.E. (2001). Description and prescription: How gender stereotypes prevent women's ascent up the organizational ladder. *Journal of Social Issues*, *57*(4), 657–74. https://doi.org/10.1111/0022-4537.00234

Isaac, C.A. (2011). A poetic representation: Women in medicine are "able to." *Qualitative Inquiry*, *17*(5), 447–51. https://doi.org/10.1177/1077800411405430

Jagsi, R., Guancial, E.A., Worobey, C.C., Henault, L.E., Chang, Y., Starr, R., …, & Hylek, E.M. (2006, Jul 20). The "gender gap" in authorship of academic medical literature – a 35-year perspective. *The New England Journal of Medicine*, *355*(3), 281–7. https://doi.org/10.1056/NEJMsa053910 Medline:16855268

Jolly, S., Griffith, K.A., DeCastro, R., Stewart, A., Ubel, P., & Jagsi, R. (2014, Mar 4). Gender differences in time spent on parenting and domestic responsibilities by high-achieving young physician-researchers. *Annals of Internal Medicine*, *160*(5), 344–53. https://doi.org/10.7326/M13-0974 Medline:24737273

Kray, L.J., Galinsky, A.D., & Thompson, L. (2002). Reversing the gender gap in negotiations: An exploration of stereotype regeneration. *Organizational Behavior and Human Decision Processes*, *87*(2), 386–410. https://doi.org/10.1006/obhd.2001.2979

Leininger, M., & McFarland, M. (2002). *Transcultural nursing: Concepts, theories and practice* (3rd ed.). New York: McGraw-Hill.

Leiter, M.P., Frank, E., & Matheson, T.J. (2009, Dec). Demands, values, and burnout: Relevance for physicians. *Canadian Family Physician Medecin de famille Canadien, 55*(12), 1225.e1–1225.e6. Medline:20008605

Levinson, W., Tolle, S.W., & Lewis, C. (1989, Nov 30). Women in academic medicine. Combining career and family. *TheNew England Journal of Medicine, 321*(22), 1511–17. https://doi.org/10.1056/NEJM198911303212205 Medline:2811971

Magrane, D., Helitzer, D., Morahan, P., Chang, S., Gleason, K., Cardinali, G., & Wu, C.C. (2012, Dec). Systems of career influences: A conceptual model for evaluating the professional development of women in academic medicine. *Journal of Women's Health (2002), 21*(12), 1244–51. https://doi.org/10.1089/jwh.2012.3638 Medline:23101486

McGuire, L.K., Bergen, M.R., & Polan, M.L. (2004). Career advancement for women faculty in a U.S. school of medicine: Perceived needs. *Academic Medicine: Journal of the Association of American Medical College, 79*(4), 319–25. https://doi.org/10.1097/00001888-200404000-00007 Medline:15044163

Mead, M. (1937). *Cooperation and competition among primitive peoples*. New York: McGraw Hill Publishing Co.

Murti, L. (2012). Who benefits from the white coat? Gender differences in occupational citizenship among Asian-Indian doctors. *Ethnic and Racial Studies, 35*(12), 2035–53. https://doi.org/10.1080/01419870.2011.631555

Nath, V., Marx, C., Lees, P., Kasaraneni, K., & Davies, S. (2014). Women in medicine: Improving women doctors' ability to achieve their full leadership potential. *BMJ, 349*. https://doi.org/10.1136/bmj.g7649

Nieman, L.Z., Foxhall, L.E., Chuang, A.Z., Cheng, L., & Prager, T.C. (2004, Jan). Evaluating the Texas Statewide Family Practice Preceptorship Program, 1992–2000. *Academic Medicine: Journal of the Association of American Medical College, 79*(1), 62–8. https://doi.org/10.1097/00001888-200401000-00014 Medline:14690999

Palepu, A., Carr, P.L., Friedman, R.H., Ash, A.S., & Moskowitz, M.A. (2000, Feb). Specialty choices, compensation, and career satisfaction of underrepresented minority faculty in academic medicine. *Academic Medicine: Journal of the Association of American Medical Colleges, 75*(2), 157–60. https://doi.org/10.1097/00001888-200002000-00014 Medline:10693848

Pololi, L.H., & Jones, S.J. (2010, Oct). Women faculty: An analysis of their experiences in academic medicine and their coping strategies. *Gender Medicine, 7*(5), 438–50. https://doi.org/10.1016/j.genm.2010.09.006 Medline:21056870

Rojas, C., Samson, S.N., Ullilen, J.F., Amoateng-Adjepong, Y., & Manthous, C.A. (2011, Jan). Are international and American graduates equally

ACGME competent? Results of a pilot study. *Connecticut Medicine, 75*(1), 31–4, quiz 35–6. Medline:21329290

Rosser, V.J. (2003). Faculty and staff members' perceptions of effective leadership: Are there differences between men and women leaders? *Equity & Excellence in Education, 36*, 71–81. https://doi.org/10.1080/10665680303501

Rudman, L.A., & Kilianski, S.E. (2000). Implicit and explicit attitudes toward female authority. *Personality and Social Psychology Bulletin, 26*(11), 1315–28. https://doi.org/10.1177/0146167200263001

Schein, V.E., Mueller, R., Lituchy, T., & Liu, J. (1996). Think manager – Think male: A global phenomenon? *Journal of Organizational Behavior, 17*(1), 33–41. https://doi.org/10.1002/(SICI)1099-1379(199601)17:1<33::AID-JOB778>3.0.CO;2-F

Schmader, T., Whitehead, J., & Wysocki, V.H. (2007). A linguistic comparison of letters of recommendation for male and female chemistry and biochemistry job applicants. *Sex Roles, 57*(7–8), 509–14. https://doi.org/10.1007/s11199-007-9291-4 Medline:18953419

Sczesny, S., Spreemann, S., & Stahlberg, D. (2006). Masculine = competent? Physical appearance and sex as sources of gender-stereotypic attributions. *Swiss Journal of Psychology, 65*(1), 15–23. https://doi.org/10.1024/1421-0185.65.1.15

Sekaquaptewa, D., & Thompson, M. (2003). Solo status, stereotype threat, and performance expectancies: Their effects on women's performance. *Journal of Experimental Social Psychology, 39*(1), 68–74. https://doi.org/10.1016/S0022-1031(02)00508-5

Shollen, S.L., Bland, C.J., Finstad, D.A., & Taylor, A.L. (2009, Jan). Organizational climate and family life: How these factors affect the status of women faculty at one medical school. *Academic Medicine: Journal of the Association of American Medical College, 84*(1), 87–94. https://doi.org/10.1097/ACM.0b013e3181900edf Medline:19116483

Taylor, K.S., Lambert, T.W., & Goldacre, M.J. (2009). Career progression and destinations, comparing men and women in the NHS: Postal questionnaire surveys. *BMJ, 338*(jun02 1), b1735. https://doi.org/10.1136/bmj.b1735 Medline:19493938

Tylor, E. (1871). *Burnett. Primitive culture: Researches into the development of mythology, philosophy, religion, art and custom*. London: Bradbury Evans and Co.

Valian, V. (1999). *Why so slow? The advancement of women*. Cambridge, MA: MIT Press.

Vinson, D.C., Paden, C., Devera-Sales, A., Marshall, B., & Waters, E.C. (1997, Dec). Teaching medical students in community-based practices: A national survey of generalist physicians. *The Journal of Family Practice*, *45*(6), 487–94. Medline:9420584

Westring, A.F., Speck, R.M., Dupuis Sammel, M., Scott, P., Conant, E.F., Tuton, L.W., …, & Grisso, J.A. (2014). Culture matters: The pivotal role of culture for women's careers in academic medicine. *Academic Medicine: Journal of the Association of American Medical College*, *89*(4), 658–63. https://doi.org/10.1097/ACM.0000000000000173 Medline:24556773

Yedidia, M.J., & Bickel, J. (2001, May). Why aren't there more women leaders in academic medicine? The views of clinical department chairs. *Academic Medicine: Journal of the Association of American Medical College*, *76*(5), 453–65. https://doi.org/10.1097/00001888-200105000-00017 Medline:11346523

4 Current State of Women in Medicine: The Statistics

DEENA M. HAMZA AND SHELLEY ROSS

Many of the chapters in *Female Doctors in Canada* refer to statistics regarding the number of positions, or lack thereof, that women hold in the medical field. These statistics may provide information on the proportion of females entering medical school compared to males, or may provide information on the proportion of females who plan to become generalists versus specialists, among other gender indicators. Regardless of the type of indicator, Canadian statistics confirm that observable gender differences exist. In some cases, disparities identified in literature are no longer accurate based on more recent information, such as differences between genders related to hours worked per week. These factors are astutely disconfirmed and presented with the most up-to-date Canadian statistics available.

This book guides the reader through various value lenses on gender differences generated by the experiences of each individual author. For example, authors discuss differences in communication styles between males and females and how this may lead to dissimilarities in patient-centred care; culture as one of many elements that may lead to barriers in advancement to leadership positions; specialty-specific medical culture and the covert exclusion of females in certain practice types, such as surgical specialties; and work-life balance as a potential barrier that significantly contributes to gender differences in medicine. Often, these accounts are paired with statistics; however, these statistics are point-in-time and context specific. Indeed, the proportions illustrated by authors need to be true to their experiences and reflective of the history of the medical environment in Canada.

As such, the purpose of this chapter is to extract pertinent ideas identified by the authors and provide the most up-to-date Canadian statistics delineated by gender, where possible, to pair candid experiences in the medical field with the current state of these differences. For ease of navigation, recurring concepts in various chapters have been combined and matched with the appropriate up-to-date information.

Summary of Themes in Women in Medicine*

- The gender distribution of the physician workforce illustrated by broad specialty
- The shift in the proportion of women entering medical school, paired with the number of medical degrees awarded
- The proportion of physicians in Canada by age and gender
- The underrepresentation of women in leadership roles
- The proportion of women practising as generalists versus specialists
- The gender distribution of physicians who are international medical graduates, by specialty
- Differences and similarities in physician work hours and practice patterns by gender
- Mistreatment during medical training based on gender, race/ethnicity, and sexual orientation

*The summary of themes that can be illustrated through Canadian statistics on the topic.

Physicians in Canada: The Workforce at a Glance

According to the Canadian Medical Association, there are 83,159 active physicians in Canada, which is approximately 2.28 physicians for every 1,000 people in the country (Canadian Medical Association [CMA], 2017). The proportion of all physicians (52% family physicians, 48% specialists in other areas) indicates that 41% of physicians are female and 59% are male; however, a greater proportion of family physicians under the age of 35 are female (64%) (CMA, 2017). Further, in 2016 53% of first-year medical students were female while 47% were male (Association of Faculties of Medicine of Canada [AFMC], 2016).

The Proportion of Women in Medical School and Degree Awardees

A recurrent theme uniting various chapters is the proportion of women entering medical school and how this rate has steadily increased from the 1940s to the estimated proportion of medical degree awardees in

2019 (Table 1, Figure 1). In the early 1940s, less than 5% of graduates with a medical doctor degree were female (Figure 1). In contrast, in 2014 approximately 58% of graduates from medical schools across Canada were female and, based on current undergraduate enrolment, this

Table 1. Proportion of females in the first year of medical school from 1957 to 2016

Year	Males	Females
Five-Year Increments		
1957/58	925	86 (8.5%)
1962/63	941	120 (11.3%)
1967/68	1,054	179 (14.5%)
1972/73	1,318	445 (25.2%)
1977/78	1,224	602 (33.0%)
1982/83	1,072	810 (43.0%)
1987/88*	929	815 (46.7%)
1992/93**	828	776 (48.4%)
1997/98	798	779 (49.5%)
2002/03	830	1,198 (59.1%)
Yearly Increments		
2007/08	1,094	1,475 (57.4%)
2008/09	1,127	1,533 (57.6%)
2009/10	1,170	1,572 (57.3%)
2010/11	1,232	1,597 (56.5%)
2011/12	1,325	1,577 (54.3%)
2012/13	1,299	1,620 (55.5%)
2013/14	1,285	1,630 (55.9%)
2014/15	1,288	1,633 (55.9%)
2015/16	1,367	1,552 (53.2%)

Source: Adapted from the Canadian Medical Association Physician Data Center: Canadian physician statistics, taken from the Office of Research of Information Services, Association of Faculties of Medicine of Canada, 2016.

* 1987/88: No students were admitted into the first year of medical school at the University of Saskatchewan.

** 1992/93: No students were admitted into the first year of medical school at the Université de Montréal.

Figure 1. Proportion of medical doctor degrees awarded by Canadian universities from 1940–2019,* by gender

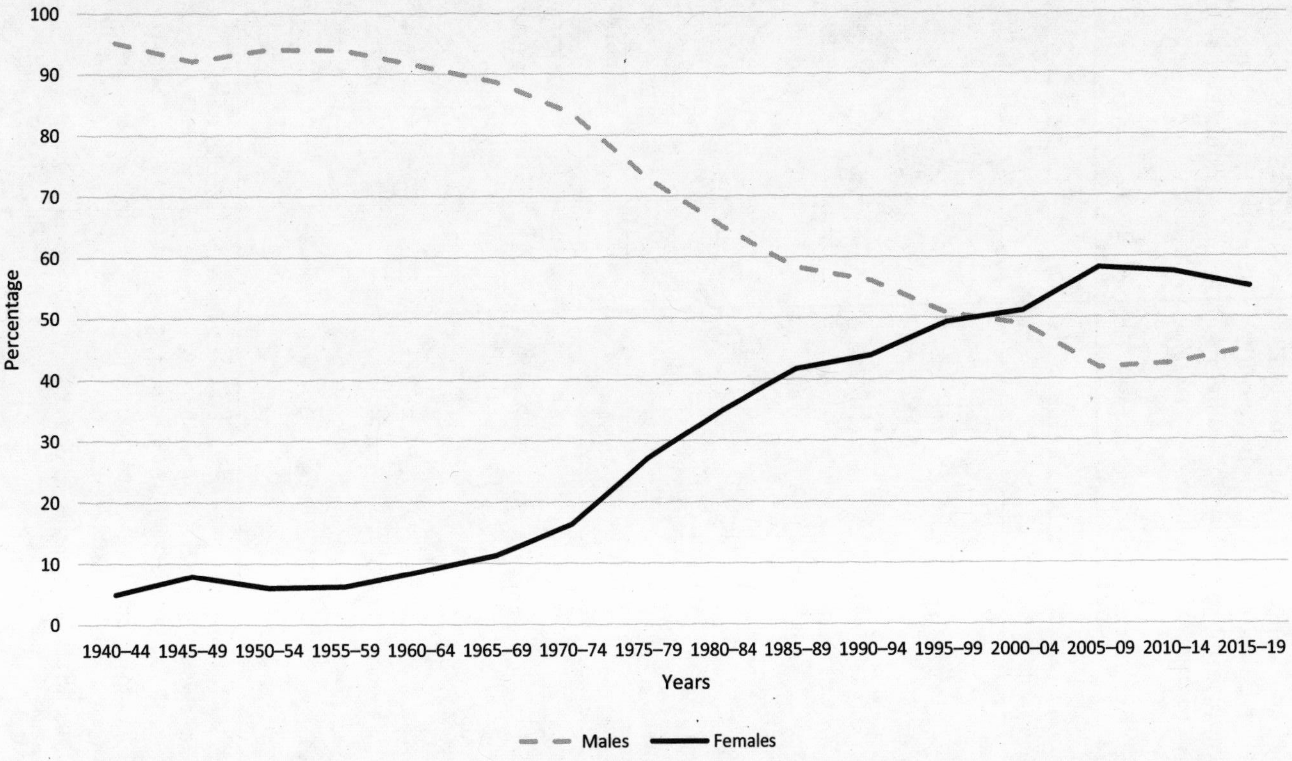

Source: Adapted from the Association of Faculties of Medicine of Canada, Canadian Medical Education Statistics 2016.

* 2019 values are based on undergraduate enrolment.

Table 2. Proportion of physicians in Canada by age and gender, in 2017

Age	Males	Females
<35	3,010 (39.5%)	4,597 (60.4%)
35–44	9,521 (48.0%)	10,309 (52.0%)
45–54	11,675 (57.0%)	8,813 (43.0%)
55–64	12,889 (64.5%)	7,105 (35.5%)
65+	10,301 (79.9%)	2,581 (20.0%)

Source: Adapted from the Canadian Medical Association Masterfile, January 2017.

proportion is expected to remain relatively constant (Figure 1). In fact, since 2000, more females were awarded medical doctor degrees than males (Figure 1). In addition, information on the greater number of practising physicians that are female and under the age of 35 (Table 2) coincides with the narrowing of the gender gap illustrated by the number of first-year medical students beginning in 1982 (Table 1). These up-to-date statistics corroborate perspectives presented in other chapters in this book that the state of medicine has changed, with greater visibility of women in the field.

The Underrepresentation of Women in Leadership Roles

The experiences shared with the reader aim to demonstrate the conundrum of gender inequalities in medicine, specifically, how the grand increase in number of females entering medicine and receiving medical degrees over time is not paired with increased visibility of females in leadership positions (Chapters 5 and 7). This underrepresentation has been examined as a reality in academic medicine in published literature (Zhuge et al., 2011, p. 5); however, there appears to be no census or Canadian retrieval of information identifying the gender distribution of full-time and part-time faculty of medicine members (Table 3)

Canadian data on the distribution of males and females in academic positions, beyond research studies and anecdotal accounts, are necessary to provide an accurate picture of gender differences now and in the future. This information is important to capture as authors discuss the implications of the underrepresentation of women in leadership positions, such as diminishing role, opinion, and insight at a policy-making level – currently, only one voice is heard.

Table 3. Proportion of faculty members in Canada in 2014/2015

Faculty of Medicine members across Canada	Faculty position	Number of members
Full-time faculty members	Professor	3,805
	Associate professor	4,033
	Assistant professor	4,896
	Instructor/other	875
	Total	13,609
Part-time faculty members	Paid	12,908
	Volunteer	25,076
	Total	37,984

Source: Adapted from the Association of Faculties of Medicine of Canada, Canadian Medical Education Statistics 2016, Table 65.

The Proportion of Women in Medical Specialties

Gender differences are also identified when observing trends in medical specialties, particularly the greater proportion of females practicing family medicine in comparison to the much smaller proportion practising a surgical specialty (Table 4). Although this appears to be the pattern of practising physicians in 2017, the gender gap seems to be closing for family medicine (Figure 2) and much more so for medical/clinical specialists (Table 5, Figure 3), laboratory medicine specialists (Table 5, Figure 4), and surgical specialists (Table 5, Figure 5) when examining the 2016 cohort entering formal medical practice and the trends in practice trainees from 2012 to 2017. Interestingly, the practice entry cohort in 2016 illustrates a new gender gap, with the underrepresentation of males in family medicine (Table 5). Authors have suggested the increased interest of females entering family medicine may be related to the ability to have flexible, plannable hours, and more patient interaction (Chapter 5).

Although the authors describe the underrepresentation of women in specialties, based on the practice entry information, it appears that the gender gap is closing. Potentially the inference is that the culture of medicine has changed, and gender gaps will continue to be minimal in the future, or another inference may be that changes occur during medical training that results in the shift in distribution of practicing

Table 4. Proportion of practising physicians in Canada in 2017, distributed by specialty and gender

Specialty	Males	Females
Family medicine/general practice	23,628 (54.7%)	19,529 (45.2%)
Medical/clinical specialists	17,011 (60.4%)	11,126 (39.5%)
Laboratory medicine specialists	1,038 (58.7%)	727 (41.1%)
Surgical specialists	7,210 (71.6%)	2,856 (28.4%)
Medical scientists	11 (100.0%)	0 (0.0%)
All physicians	48,898 (58.8%)	34,238 (41.2%)

Source: Adapted from Canadian Medical Association Masterfile, January 2017.

Table 5. Proportion of practice entry cohort (exiting trainees) in Canada in 2016, by specialty and gender

Specialty	Male	Female
Family medicine	436 (37.9%)	715 (62.1%)
Medical specialties	633 (45.9%)	746 (54.1%)
Laboratory medicine specialties	40 (54.1%)	34 (45.9%)
Surgical specialties	279 (55.7%)	222 (44.3%)

Source: Adapted from the 2017 Canadian Post-M.D. Education Registry, data table H-7.

physicians by specialty. Statistics for the 2017 practice entry cohort will be available soon and may provide further insight on this observed change in the gender gap.

The Proportion of Women Who Are International Medical Graduates Completing Post-Medical Degree Training in Canada

It has been suggested that there are barriers faced by individuals who complete their medical education in a foreign country and come to Canada for postgraduate medical training (Chapter 6). These barriers include the preconceived notion that international medical graduates (IMGs) are not as competent as Canadian graduates, and this discrimination is suggested to be more prominent in some specialties (such as surgery) than others. The authors also describe how race and ethnicity

Figure 2. Proportion of post-medical degree trainees in family medicine in Canada from 2012–2017, by gender

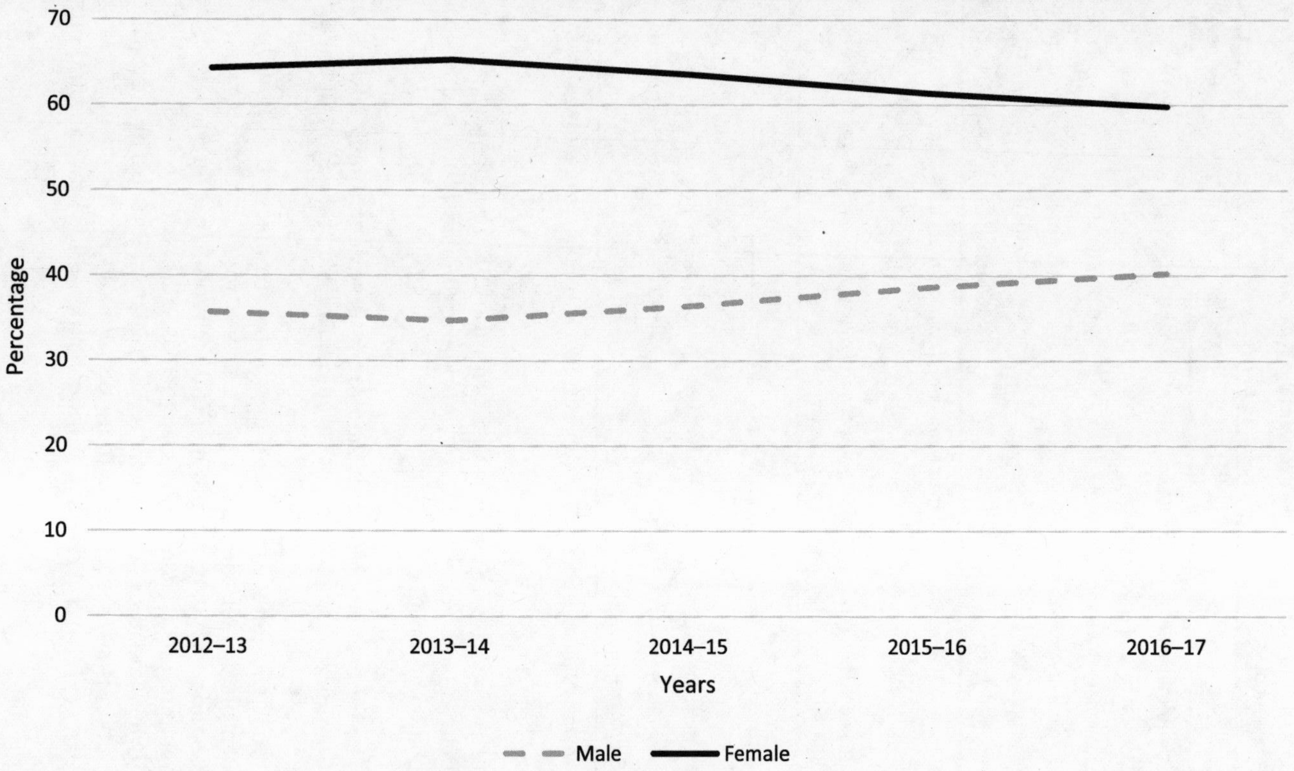

Source: Adapted from the 2017 Canadian Post-MD Education Registry, data Table 1-3

Figure 3. Proportion of post-medical degree trainees in medical specialities* in Canada from 2012–2017, by gender

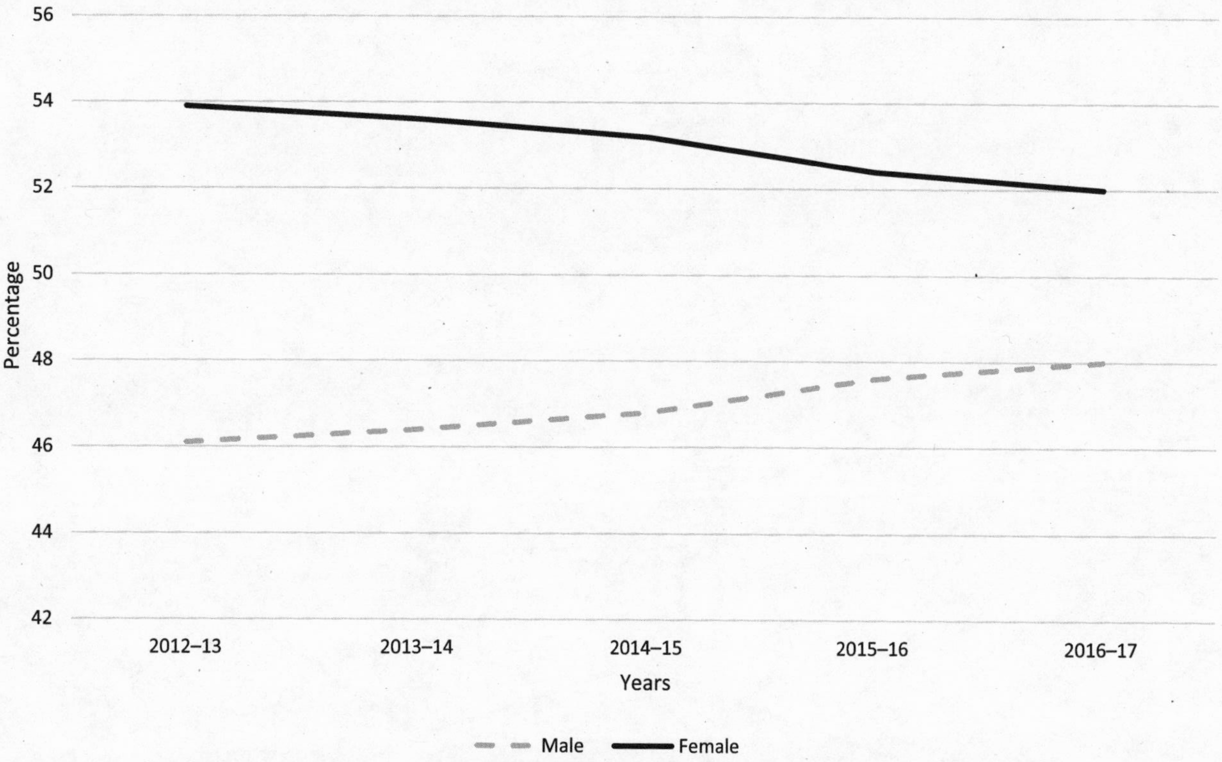

Source: Adapted from the 2017 Canadian Post-M.D. Education Registry, data Table 1-3

*Medical specialties include anaesthesiology, public health/preventive medicine, dermatology, diagnostic radiology, emergency medicine, internal medicine, medical genetics, neurology, nuclear medicine, palliative medicine, pediatrics, physical medicine and rehabilitation, psychiatry, and radiation oncology.

Figure 4. Proportion of post-medical degree trainees in laboratory medicine specialties* in Canada from 2012–2017, by gender

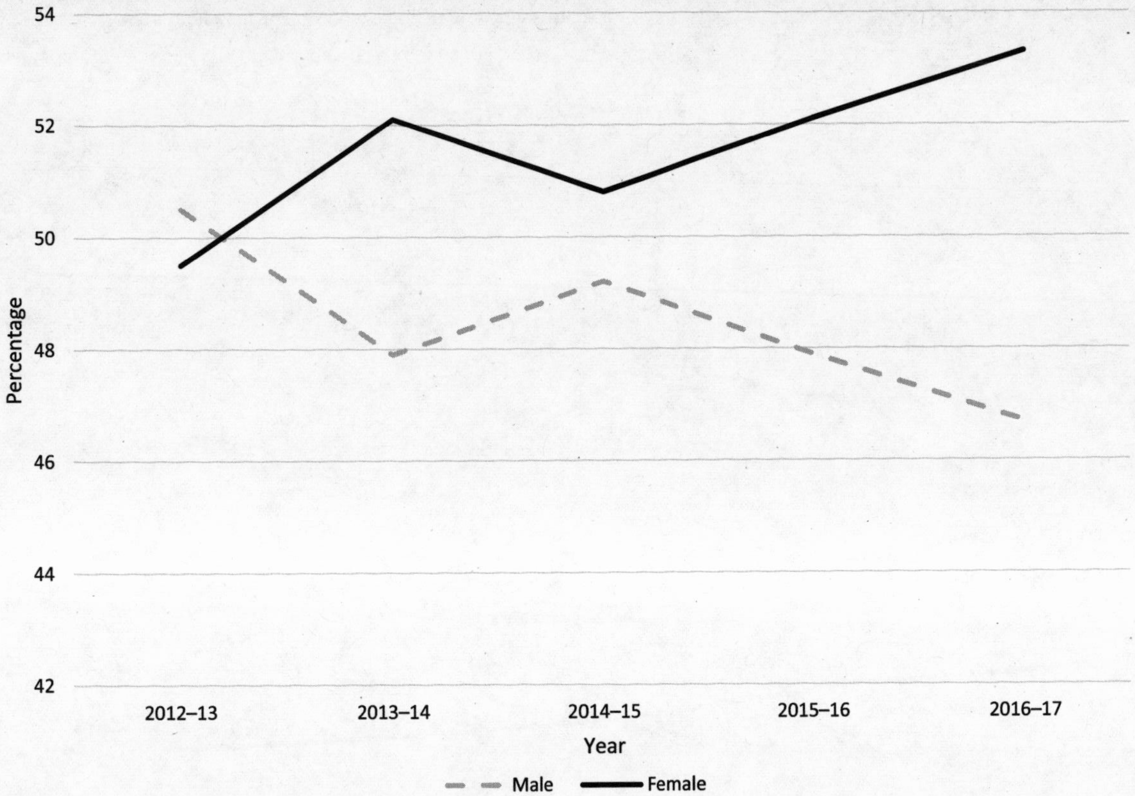

Source: Adapted from the 2017 Canadian Post-M.D. Education Registry, data Table 1-3

*Laboratory medicine specialties include anatomical pathology, general pathology, hematological pathology, medical biochemistry, medical microbiology, and neuropathology.

Figure 5. Proportion of post-medical education trainees in surgical specialties* in Canada from 2012–2017, by gender

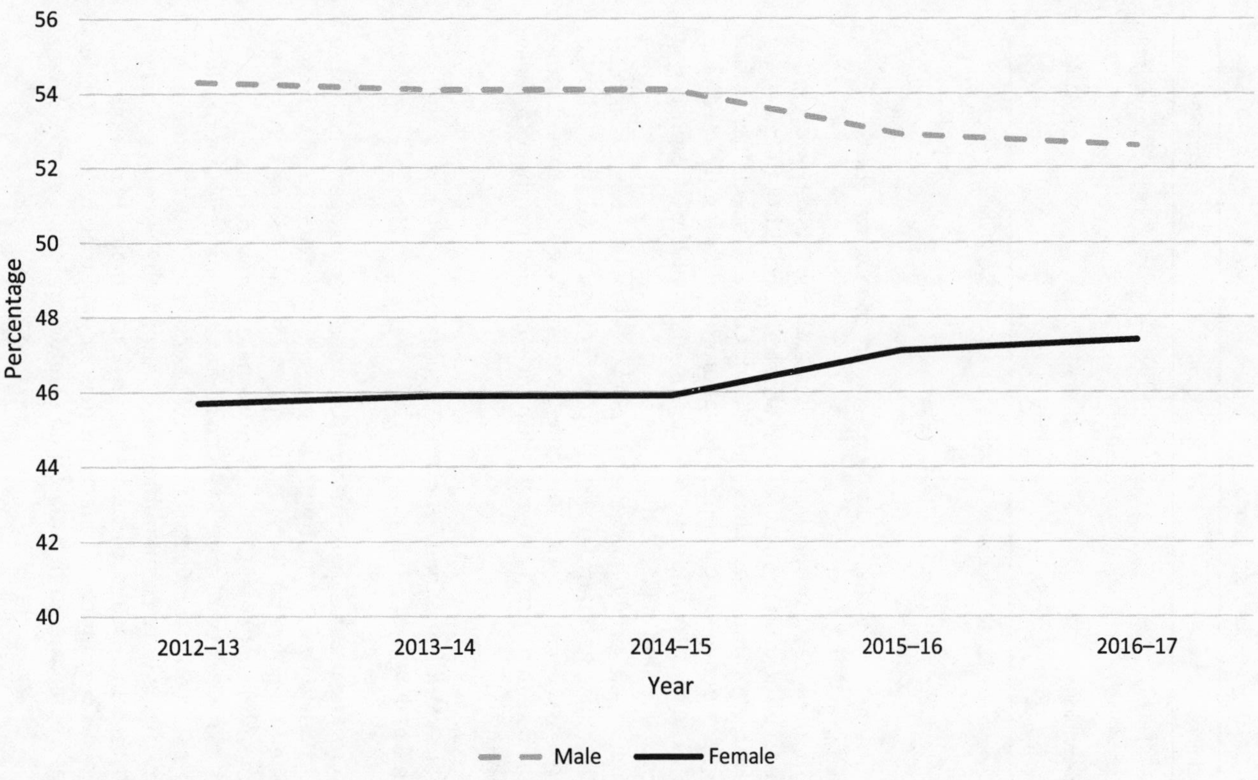

Source: Adapted from the 2017 Canadian Post-M.D. Education Registry, data Table 1-3

* Surgical specialties include cardiac surgery, general surgery, vascular surgery, neurosurgery, obstetrics/gynecology, ophthalmology, otolaryngology – head and neck surgery, orthopedic surgery, plastic surgery, and urology.

Table 6. International medical graduates completing post-medical degree training in Canada in 2015, by specialty and gender

Field of training	Males	Females
Family medicine	241 (45.0%)	294 (55.0%)
Medical specialties	1,650 (57.7%)	1,209 (42.3%)
Laboratory medicine	76 (38.6%)	121 (61.4%)
Surgical specialties	727 (77.8%)	207 (22.2%)

Source: Canadian Post-MD Education Registry, the National IMG Database Report, 2017.

amplifies the existing discrimination women encounter when training and when practising medicine.

In 2015, the largest proportion of IMGs had undertaken postgraduate medical education in medical and surgical specialties, followed by family and laboratory specialties (Table 6). Of these specialties, more females than males were training in laboratory and family medicine (Table 6). The greatest underrepresentation of female IMGs is observed for surgical specialties (Table 6).

As mentioned previously, the authors present evidence suggesting that females gravitate to specific practices based on the ability to maintain a work-life balance and integrate family obligations. Future Canadian research in this area will provide clearer insight into these observations.

Comparing Work Hours and Practice Patterns between Genders

Work hours and practice patterns are two broad themes described by the authors in Chapters 5, 7, and, 8 with the suggestion that female physicians contribute less hours per week to the physician workforce and spend more time with patients. On average, female family physicians work 45 hours per week compared to 49 hours by their male counterparts – a 4 hour per week difference (Figure 6). Specialists in areas other than family medicine have comparable work hours with 48 hours per week reported by females, and 51 hours per week by males – a 3 hour per week difference (Figure 6). In fact, the gender gap in hours worked per week has changed significantly when examining trends from 1982 to

Figure 6. Average hours worked per week by physicians in Canada in 2014, distributed by gender and broad specialty

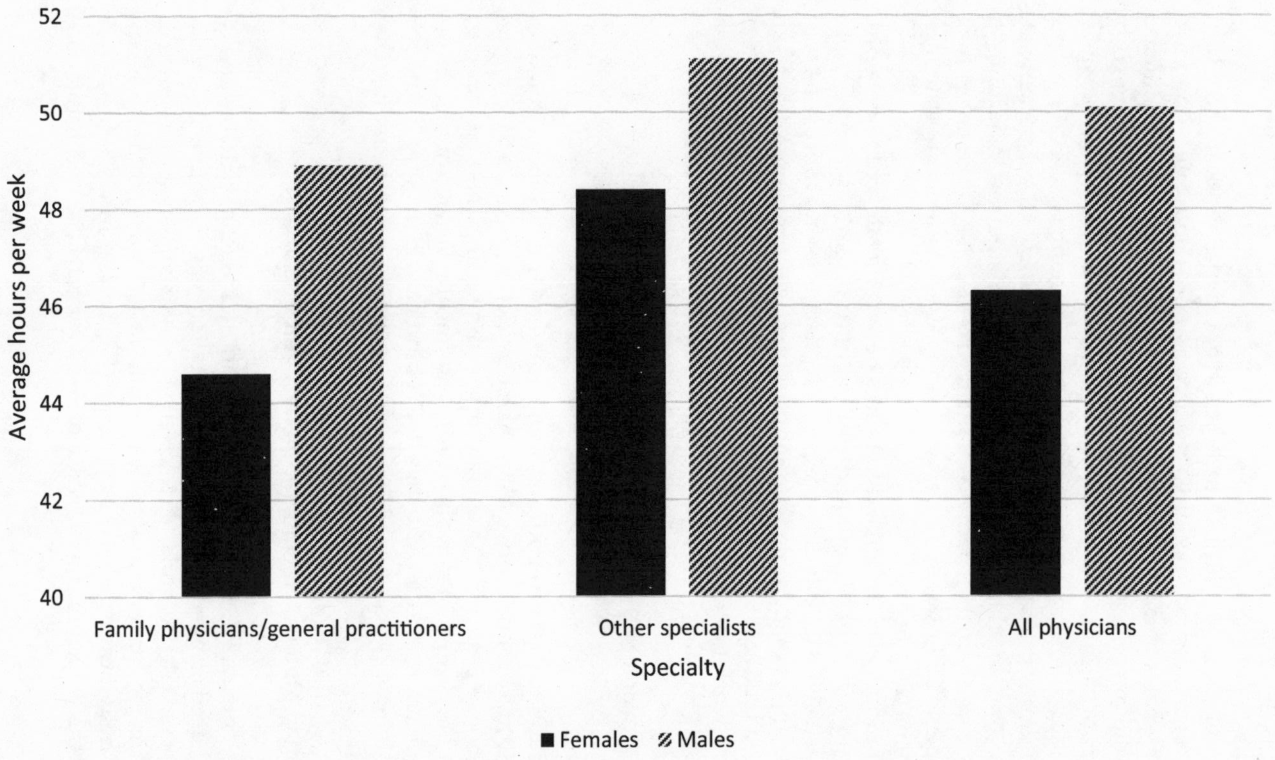

Source: Adapted from the 2014 National Physician Survey by the College of Family Physicians of Canada, Canadian Medical Association, and the Royal College of Physicians and Surgeons of Canada

2014 in which both male and female physicians are contributing similar work hours per week (Figure 7).

In addition to similarities in hours worked per week by all physicians, regardless of specialty, practice patterns indicate similarities between males and females. More specifically, both males and females spend the majority of their time engaging with patients, followed by direct patient care, and teaching responsibilities (Figure 8); however, the gender differences may not be as great as in the past. For example, males work less than three hours more per week in direct patient care and less than one hour more in teaching responsibilities in addition to patient care than their female counterparts (Figure 8). Female physicians spend 1.5 hours more per week on indirect patient care than male physicians (Figure 8).

The authors also describe differences between male and female physicians in terms of quality and productivity of patient care (Chapter 7). It has been suggested that female physicians spend more time with patients and provide a higher quality of care, while male physicians are more productive and provide care to a greater number of patients during their work hours. Currently, this is an avenue for future examination on a Canadian level.

The Proportion of Physicians in Patient Care Settings, by Gender

In addition to practice patterns, there are gender differences in patient care setting chosen by physicians. Some evidence suggests that women often choose group practices over other care settings and are overrepresented in community health centres and health service organizations (Chapter 10). Canadian statistics in 2014 indicate that a greater proportion of female physicians (33%) are practising in a group setting than male physicians (25%) (Figure 9).

Comparing Mode of Remuneration between Genders

Beyond potential differences in work hours and practice patterns of physicians based on gender, mode of remuneration may also have observable differences. For example, 42% of male physicians receive remuneration from fee-for-service activities, while this mode accounts for only 35% of activities by female physicians (Figure 10). In addition, female physicians engage in more blended (44% versus 42%) and capitation/

Figure 7. Trends in average hours worked per week by physicians from 1982–2014, distributed by gender

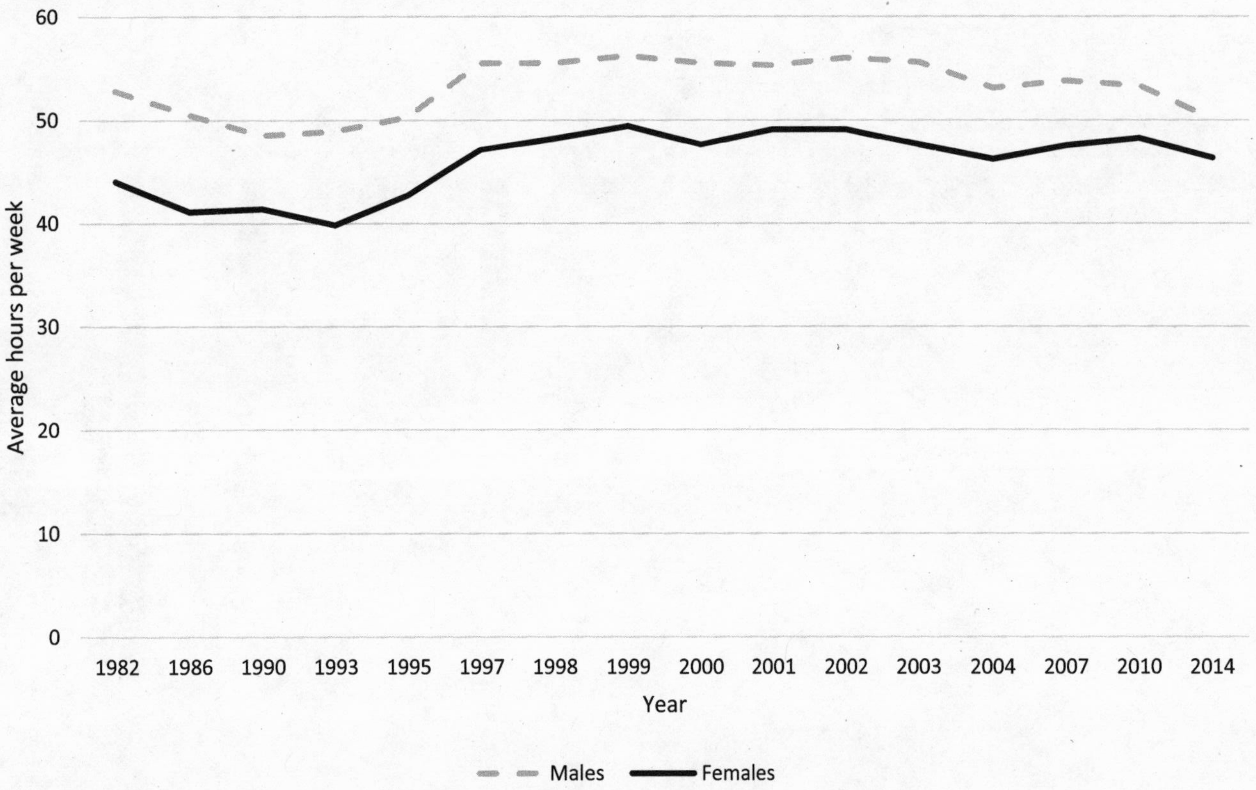

Source: Adapted from the National Physician Survey 1982–2014. Surveys before 1994 and after 2004 reflect census responses from all active physicians in Canada. Surveys in the 1993–2003 iterations were based on a sample of active physicians in Canada.

Figure 8. Average hours worked per week by physicians attributed to specific tasks, distributed by gender

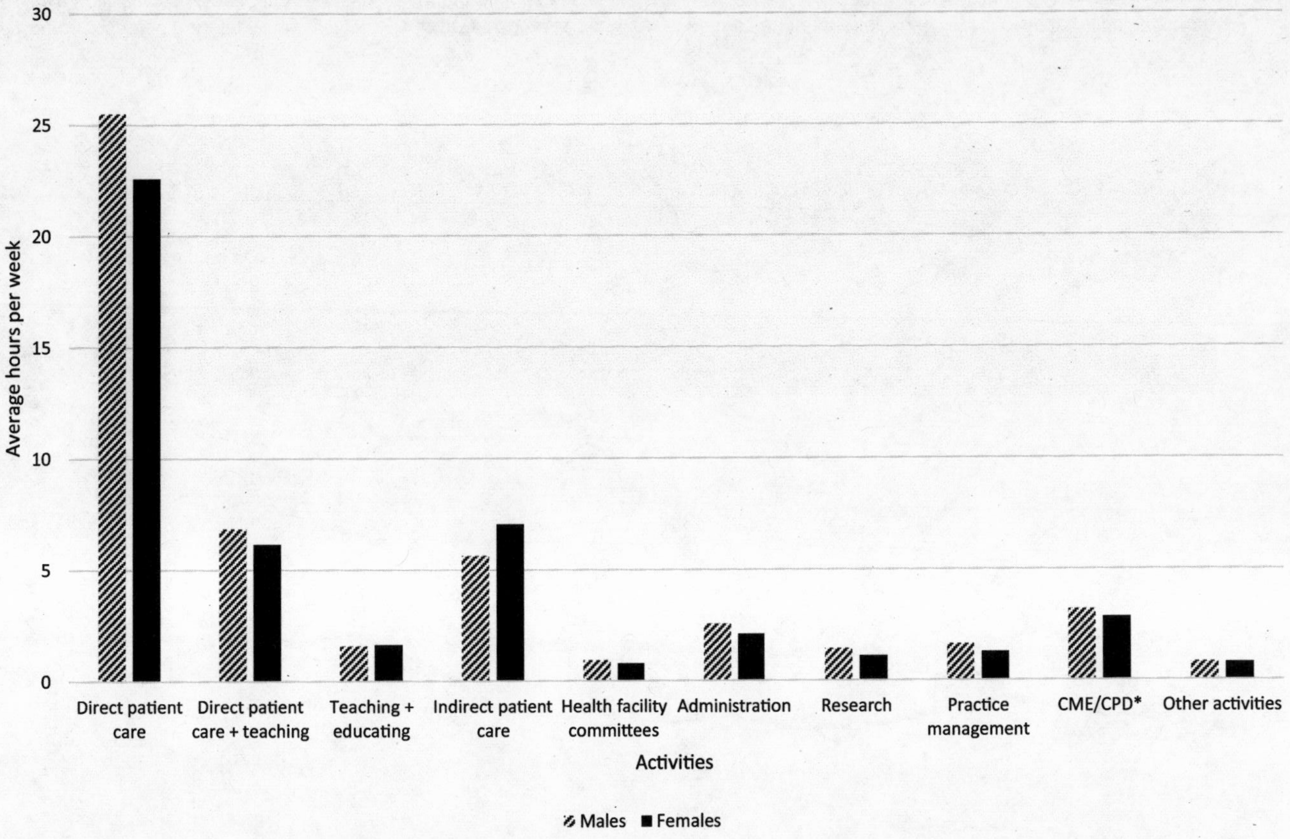

Source: Adapted from the 2014 National Physician Survey by the College of Family Physicians of Canada, Canadian Medical Association, and the Royal College of Physicians and Surgeons of Canada

* CME = continuing medical education; CPD = continuing professional development

Figure 9. Proportion of physicians by main patient care setting and gender in Canada in 2014

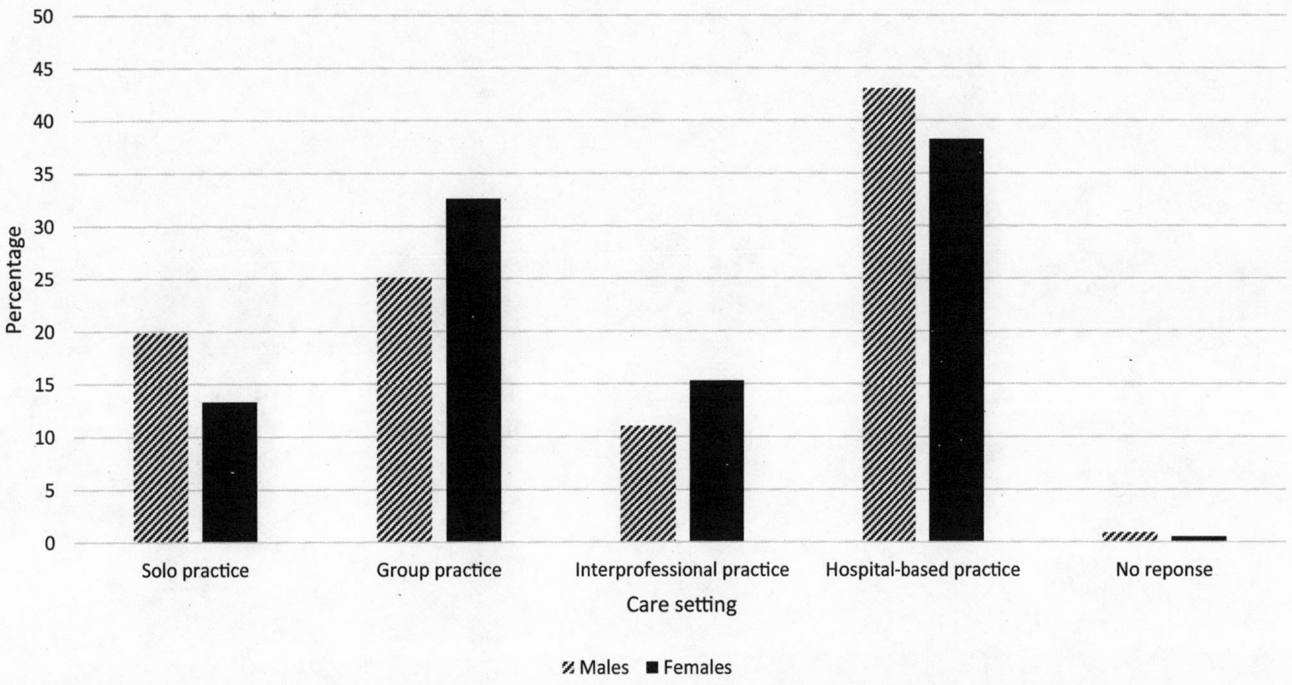

Source: Adapted from the National Physician Survey, 2014, by the College of Family Physicians of Canada, Canadian Medical Association, and the Royal College of Physicians and Surgeons of Canada

Figure 10. Proportion of physicians by mode of remuneration and gender in Canada in 2013

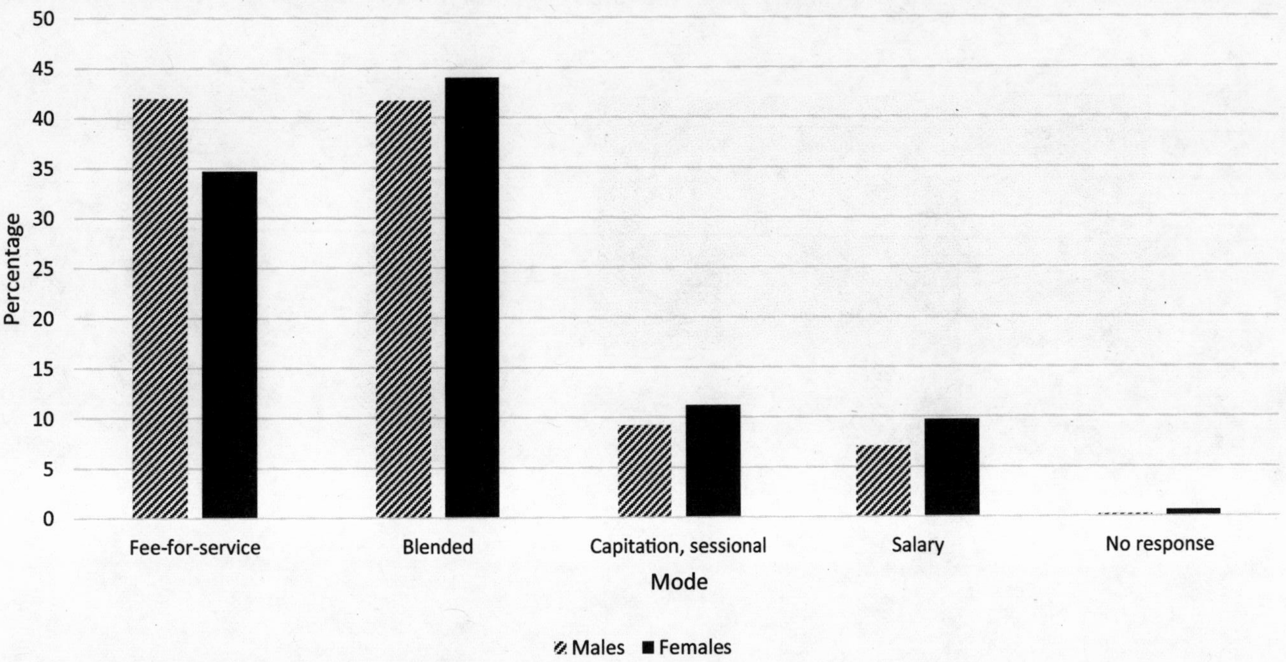

Source: Adapted from National Physician Survey, 2013, by the College of Family Physicians of Canada, Canadian Medical Association, and the Royal College of Physicians and Surgeons of Canada.

Each category represents 90% or more of professional earnings from that mode.

Figure 11. Proportion of family physicians by mode of remuneration and gender in Canada in 2013

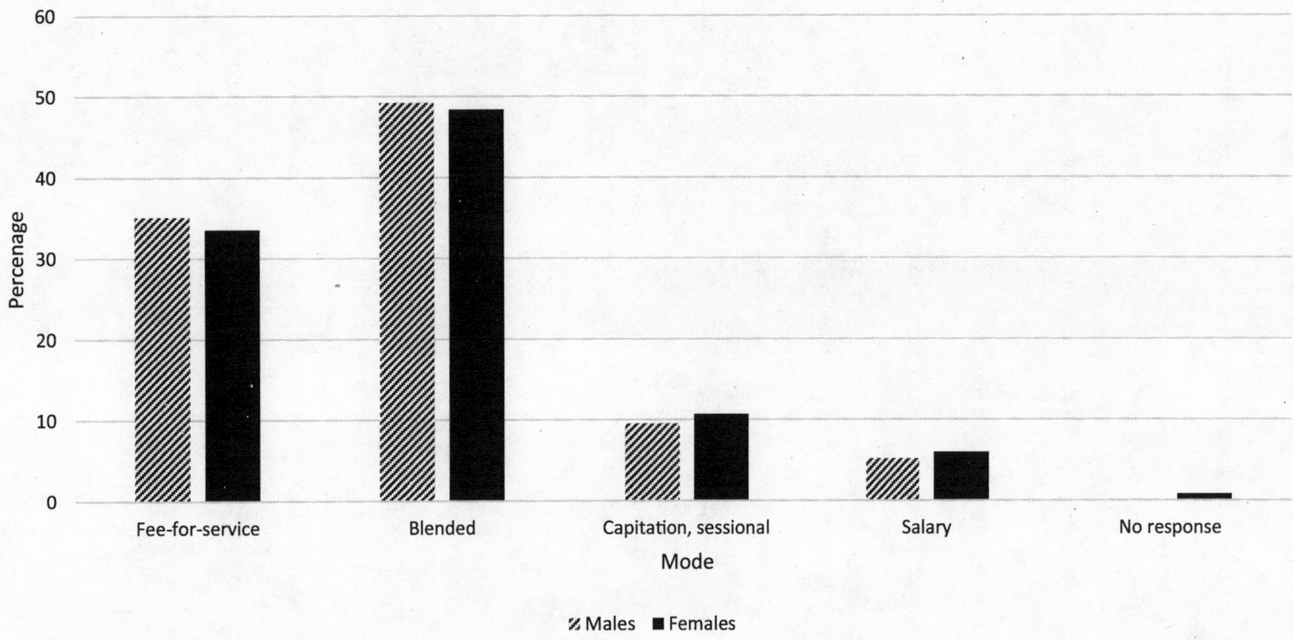

Source: Adapted from National Physician Survey, 2013 by the College of Family Physicians of Canada, Canadian Medical Association, and the Royal College of Physicians and Surgeons of Canada

Each category represents 90% or more of professional earnings from that mode.

sessional opportunities (11% versus 9%), and receive more remuneration by salary (10% versus 7%) than male physicians (Figure 10).

Chapter 3 describes the mode of remuneration for family physicians, specifically, identifying that more than 50% of compensation is from sources outside of fee-for-service activities. This is confirmed with Canadian statistics from 2013 indicating that both male and female physicians received most of their compensation from blended opportunities (Figure 11). Interestingly, there are small gender differences in the mode of remuneration for family physicians (Figure 11).

Mistreatment during Medical Training

Findings from published literature and experiences from authors present the reality some women face during medical school in the form of mistreatment as a consequence of gender (Chapter 3, 5, and 10). The graduation questionnaire administered across Canada by the Association of Faculties of Medicine of Canada has captured this information, including mistreatment as a result of other factors; however, this information is not categorized by gender. Although this book focuses on the experiences of women, the information captured on mistreatment is too important to be overlooked. As such, genderless information is presented in this section, with the recommendation for future opportunities to delineate experiences of mistreatment by gender.

A consistent increase from 2015 to 2017 is noted for trainees who experienced withheld opportunities for training and rewards; were subject to sexist remarks or names; and received lower evaluations or grades as a result of their gender (Table 7). A consistent, but cautiously interpreted, increase is also noted for trainees experiencing public humiliation during medical school from 28% in 2015 to 44% in 2017 (Table 7).

An increase in trainees experiencing mistreatment as a result of race or ethnicity is also noted from 2015 to 2017, specifically related to withheld opportunities for training and rewards; offensive remarks or names; and lower evaluations or grades (Table 7).

Denial of training opportunities and rewards, and receiving lower evaluations or grades as a result of sexual orientation is observed to have increased from 2016 to 2016 (Table 7). A slight decrease in offensive remarks or names based on sexual orientation is also observed (Table 7).

Table 7. Proportion of medical trainees experiencing mistreatment from faculty, nurses, residents/interns, employees/staff, and other students during medical school in Canada in 2017 (does not include mistreatment from patients and their families)

	2015		2016		2017	
Behaviour	No (%)	Yes (%)	No (%)	Yes (%)	No (%)	Yes (%)
Publicly humiliated*	71.4	28.3	70.7	29.3	55.9	44.1
Threatened with physical harm	97.6	2.4	97.4	2.6	98.1	1.9
Physically harmed	98.3	1.7	98.6	1.5	98.4	1.6
Required to perform personal services	87.5	12.4	85.7	14.4	89.3	10.7
Subjected to unwanted sexual advances	94.0	6.0	95.2	4.8	93.7	6.3
Asked to exchange sexual favours for grades/other rewards	99.5	0.5	99.9	0.1	99.8	0.2
Denied training/rewards based on gender	91.1	9.0	90.9	9.1	90.1	10.0
Subjected to sexist remarks/names	84.0	16.1	79.7	20.3	79.9	20.3
Received lower evaluations/grades based on gender	96.6	3.4	97.2	2.9	95.7	4.4
Denied training/rewards based on race/ethnicity	98.1	1.9	97.5	2.5	97.3	2.7
Subjected to racially/ethnically offensive remarks/names	92.4	7.6	91.5	8.6	90.5	9.5
Received lower evaluations/grades because of race/ethnicity rather than performance	98.6	1.5	98.7	1.3	98.2	1.7
Denied training/rewards based on sexual orientation	99.1	0.9	99.6	0.4	99.4	0.7

(Continued)

Table 7. Continued

	2015		2016		2017	
Subjected to offensive remarks/ names based on sexual orientation	97.7	2.3	97.2	2.7	97.8	2.1
Received lower evaluations/grades based on sexual orientation	99.4	0.6	99.7	0.3	99.5	0.6
Total	N/A	N/A	N/A	N/A	40.4	59.6

Source: Adapted from the Association of Faculties of Medicine of Canada Graduation Questionnaire, National Report 2017.

*In the 2017 iteration, "publicly embarrassed" was not included in the AFMC graduation questionnaire leading to a higher number of responses in the "publicly humiliated" category. Caution should be taken when comparing to early iterations of the questionnaire.

Although the mistreatment of medical trainees is not categorized by gender, capturing Canadian experiences provides insight into inappropriate and unacceptable challenges medical residents may face during their training. Currently, conclusions cannot be drawn regarding the proportion of females who encounter harassment and discrimination in relation to males; however, this evidence alone allows for a conscious discussion of trainee experiences and the need for improvements in the culture of medicine from students to faculty and others in leadership positions.

Summary

This chapter has summarized the current available statistics on a wide variety of issues and conceptions explored in this book. We are aware of the limitations of measuring cultural trends solely by means of a numerical analysis, and it is important to keep that in mind when weighing their significance. Moreover, the chapter must be placed in the context of the several points made by the chapter authors. In that way, the overall significance of these statistics can provide another window on the phenomenon and the role of Canadian women in medicine.

REFERENCES

Association of Faculties of Medicine of Canada. (2016). *Canadian medical education statistics.* Ottawa: Author.

Canadian Medical Association. (2017). Basic physician facts. Ottawa: Author.

Zhuge, Y., Kaufman, J., Simeone, D.M., Chen, H., & Velazquez, O.C. (2011, Apr). Is there still a glass ceiling for women in academic surgery? *Annals of Surgery, 253*(4), 637–43. https://doi.org/10.1097/SLA.0b013e3182111120 Medline:21475000

SECTION TWO

Navigating the Reality of Becoming and Being a Female Physician in a Traditionally Male Profession: Social and Cultural Issues

Most Canadians assume that for those people fortunate enough to gain admission to medical school, the greatest demands to be faced are achieving the high academic standards of the training program. In addition, while some medical school selection processes might include an expectation that candidates provide evidence of their personal ability to handle the pressures of a rigorous process, it is usually assumed that those students who are unable to withstand such studies will be winnowed out at interview time. The biggest assumption is that all medical students will be equally trained. What is often unspoken, however, is a medical culture that has been generated with certain gender assumptions. Successful female applicants to medical schools may well not comprehend how these cultural assumptions play a role in both their experiences within medical school and further training, and their experiences as they progress through their careers.

In this section, both authors examine primarily the experiences of female physicians during training, addressing two distinct but related issues that shed light on some of the barriers faced by women as they pursue medical training and plan their medical careers. In Chapter 5, Cheri Bethune presents a unique perspective on the educational and career challenges of female medical students and physicians by blending her own experience with a review of the literature in this area. In Chapter 6, Inge Schabort presents an overview of the further cultural and social challenges faced by female international medical graduates (those who pursued medical training outside Canada and want to practise in Canada) in the words of those women themselves.

5 Gendered Experience, Role Models and Mentorship, Leadership, and the Hidden Curriculum

CHERI BETHUNE

Personal story:

> *I really don't know what to do! ... I came into medicine because I thought I could make a difference ... now I really wonder if that is possible or if I should even be here at all! How did you survive it? You are courageous, outspoken, successful – a great teacher. How is it you survived the constant eye rolls, the putdowns, the sighs of exasperation? I'm getting tired of being the only one to make comments when the prof tells crude, sexist jokes about women generally or women physicians or even women as patients! Let alone the reaction of my classmates who seem tired of me ... avoid me even and brand me as a Feminist disturber! Does it get any better? Does anyone really care? I really thought that medicine was going to be so exciting, learning so much, given so much opportunity. Now I can hardly wait to get out of here.*

If this story sounds familiar, either as your own journey or that of students or colleagues you have tried to support and counsel, then this chapter is for you.

The purpose of this chapter is to enumerate the major barriers that have been well identified and persistent, and to describe the impact they have on women physicians in their professional identity formation, on their career choices, and on leadership for future generations of students and the health care system.

Introduction

There are significant barriers to women physicians having complete engagement in the practice, teaching, and being leaders in medicine.

These barriers are historic and structural, and persist despite many years of awareness. Resistance to change calls for reform (Sklar, 2016). Medicine and medical education as an organization is an "inequality regime" (Acker, 1990) that has been forged over the last century on a model of white male heterosexual identity. As a regime, it is very resistant to change as it is invisible to those who hold power and privilege within the organization and threatens loss of that very privilege if changed. These barriers have been clearly articulated for over 30 years but have persisted despite the sexes having achieved numerical equity many years ago (Association of Faculties of Medicine of Canada [AFMC], 2016).

Some might attribute these barriers to the hidden curriculum. Some would argue this has been a major excuse for failure to address their persistence. If we keep calling it hidden, then we are at risk of disavowing responsibility for it. Through articulation of the ample evidence it will be clear that these barriers are "NEON" (J. Konkin, personal communication, 2014), not hidden, and are pervasive educational issues (MacLeod, 2011).

What Are the Barriers?

1. Gendered Experience

According to Acker, to say that an organization is gendered is to suggest that "advantage, disadvantage, exploitation and control, action, and emotion, meaning and identity, are patterned through and in terms of a distinction between male and female, masculine and feminine" (Acker, 1990, p. 146).

The issues of sexual abuse and harassment in medical education are considered some of the most egregious behaviours in the faculty. Babaria et al. (2012) have shown that these issues are both pervasive and current, with more than 80% of students reporting some experience of abuse or harassment during their training. This experience appears so universal that it almost suggests that it is the norm for women medical students. However, they do not report these experiences to anyone in the medical education regime. Rather than report, they find strategies to avoid offensive behaviour or they remove themselves from the situation. Not reporting likely perpetuates the transgressions and the culture and itself becomes part of the culture. Why women do not report has many interpretations, but likely the major indictment for our medical education community, as in our communities at large, is the belief that nothing will be done. Women fear reprisal not only from the perpetrators of this abuse and harassment, but also from their classmates who they perceive will react negatively to their protests. They choose to be "good girls" and in our Western culture good girls do not speak up about these matters (Wear et al., 2007). The strategy Wear and her colleagues uncovered in their research was "to submit, don't complain, don't report" and ultimately "suck it up" (p. 23). The driving force behind this tough-minded approach is the potential impact on evaluations, which female students perceive as vulnerable to alteration – particularly the subjective comments provided by clinical supervisors. The other factors include team loyalty where harassment and abuse allegations would "ruffle feathers" or be "raising a stir" (p. 23) and would label the reporting student as one who is not a team player. This has reverberations throughout the team and speaks to a culture that has strong morals built on loyalty and submission. Added to this is the personal implications of reporting, which is construed as a weakness and, in the culture of medicine, is antithetical to the model of the capable physician. This means that women in medicine have experiences based on their gender that are different from male students (Hill & Vaughan, 2013; Phillips & Clarke, 2012).

2. Gendered Curriculum

The curriculum at both the formal and the informal level has numerous examples of how women are portrayed. The content of teaching material in most curricula continues to portray women as vulnerable and troublesome patients, and issues that might identify women as having important and unique health care issues are avoided. Even in our most sophisticated simulation teaching labs, the generic model of a male resuscitation victim (Stan the man) is the standard model for education, the male physiology and anatomy being the norm (Cheng & Yang, 2015) with scant attention to the possibility of a woman patient. Women and their presence in the educational curricula are often either ignored or presented as complicated (Phillips & Clarke, 2012; Babaria et al., 2012).

This problem extends beyond the curriculum and stereotyping of women to classroom teaching, where derogatory comments about women and women physicians are witnessed. Not only do students hear these comments but they also see them enacted when their male classmates treat women lecturers differentially through disrespectful behaviour and aggressive challenges to the content of their lecture. This is so pervasive that women report sympathy and embarrassment for their women professors (Phillips & Clarke, 2012).

Babaria et al. (2011) created a taxonomy of the pre-clinical gender-related experiences of students. She and her colleagues documented the behaviour of students, instructors, and the institution and described the emotional impact and the negative and positive adaptive strategies that women students reported to allow them to cope with their experiences. The research also documented the impact these experiences had on their future education, professional identity formation, and career path. "All of the participants in our study reported recurrent exposures to a consistent set of behaviours and attitudes that diminished the role of women in medicine" and many more subtle experiences that are often not recognized, reported or addressed (Babaria et al., 2011, p. 257; Frost & Regehr, 2013; Smith et al., 2018). It seems clear that there is a need to pay greater attention to both the overt and the subtle impact of gender-based occurrences in medical education.

These experiences of sexual harassment and gendered discrimination with the tendency to non-report can have huge consequences for the women themselves, their self-esteem and mental health, and their professional identity formation (Blanch et al., 2008; Phillips, 2009; Phillips & Clarke, 2012). This must be viewed not only at the individual level but more broadly in an environment that permits these experiences to continue, conferring a legitimacy within medicine such that it becomes the culture, impervious to change. Much like the Canadian military and other male hegemonic and hierarchical institutions, without a declaration of zero tolerance, the behaviour becomes an acceptable and perhaps even anticipated part of the culture (National Defence and the Canadian Armed Forces, 2017).

A gendered curriculum has both emotional and educational consequences for women and likely for men, particularly those who are not of the privileged white minority (Razack et al., 2015).

3. Role Models, Communities of Practice, and Career Trajectories

Role-modelling is a major factor in professional identity formation (PIF). Role models have been described as essential in PIF and are perhaps more important for women than men. A study by Lockwood & Kunda (1997) examining the impact of role models suggested that the best type of role model is someone with whom the viewer identifies. This concept is called "identity compatibility" and incorporates the feeling of belonging (Rosenthal et al., 2013, p. 464). Membership in a group is described by Wenger (1998) in his work about "communities of practice." This process begins with the novice expressing interest in the group or discipline. The group itself wields power by welcoming the novice through invitation to peripheral participation. The novice becomes involved in the group process, first through observation, then through gradual assumption or delegation of responsibilities. This is a dynamic process of initiation whereby the novice observes and then imitates the members of the group, acting more like a group member as the novices demonstrate a willingness to embrace group values. The group responds favourably by awarding the novice with greater responsibility and opportunity to learn. The novice is embraced by the community.

From an educational perspective "communities of practice" are mechanisms of apprenticeship and students gain support and opportunity through the group embracing them as protégées. In medicine, communities of practice function as learning communities, allowing continued professional development in a synergistic way. The alternative perspective is that the learning community is also a gatekeeper of who is allowed into the community. This function serves to protect the community and maintain power over membership (Hill & Vaughan, 2013; Hill et al., 2014). Students learn how to navigate their way through the complex task of acceptance into communities of practice. Male medical students seem to understand this process better than women students, and that in itself suggests that the mechanism is gendered. Male medical students are much more likely to find mentors and participate early and readily in actions that begin their early membership in learning communities (Levine et al., 2013; Hill et al., 2014; Stamm & Buddeberg-Fischer, 2011). Women students recognize that their male peers seem to gain admission to processes that are somewhat mystifying to the women. Also, they observe, the men know how to talk to the men in those communities, having conversations about shared interests outside of medicine – small talk that appears to help the men in the establishment of relationships. This includes the inclusion in camaraderie of going for a beer or playing golf outside of regular work hours. Because these disciplines are largely male dominated, it makes sense that the welcoming of newcomers would be far easier for students of a similar characteristic (Hill & Vaughan, 2013; Hill et al., 2014).

Women not only don't know how to navigate into these communities but may feel excluded if they do so because they don't share the language and articulated interests of the dominant stakeholders in those disciplines. Instead, the communities where women find themselves more comfortable and at home are those that include women, thus the perpetuation of the historic gendered career pathways of surgery for men and pediatrics and family medicine for women (Alers et al., 2014; Smith et al., 2018).

Even in disciplines such as internal medicine, where women are members but in a minority, women students observe that their role models are uninspiring. They comment on the perceived lack of respect for women team members and the deferential behaviour the women display. Students see the women on the team as minor players in a male-dominant group. On the other hand, they also express disappointment with women who act more like their male colleagues. This double standard has been articulated clearly in a study that explores the dilemma women face in a culture that has very strong gender expectations (Dolishny & Noelle, 2012). Women students expect, on the one hand, that women faculty will demonstrate strong feminine characteristics such as empathy, yet are perturbed when they hold little power or influence in their male-dominated team.

Moulton and colleagues (2013) observe that in the discipline of surgery the lack of role models, sexism, and feelings of dis-identification are pervasive and have a negative impact on women students' self-efficacy. They argue that the number of role models is inconsequential if those role models have assumed male gendered characteristics. This creates quite a conundrum as women embrace those masculine qualities to gain admission to the exclusive community of surgery. Yet this fails to shift the dominant gendered model of who and what a surgeon is for future students and for the evolution of the discipline (*British Medical Journal*, 2016).

In a medical career path, the concept of seeing oneself in the discipline is postulated as the mechanism by which students make career decisions. This "paradigmatic trajectory" is the visible career path provided by the community that shapes how individuals find meaning. This trajectory is the "most influential factor in the shaping of the learning of newcomers," and is the key focus in building the bridge between identity and practice (Moulton et al., 2013). Hill and Vaughan, (2013) divide this experience into seeing, hearing, doing, and imagining. In surgery women feel like outsiders. They see who and what surgery involves and feel they do not belong. They hear stories from others about surgical careers that do not speak of women and do not resonate with their own personal attributes. They are restricted from participation in surgical activities and skills, resulting in either no or more resoundingly negative feedback about their abilities and thus cannot imagine themselves as surgeons. This describes the trajectory that restricts women physicians' career choice (Hill & Giles, 2014; Moulton et al., 2013).

An interesting phenomenon occurs when students observe all-female teams, whether in a traditionally male defined discipline or not. Here they observe women role models differently and remark on the dynamic of the team in which they feel "at home" or "more able to be themselves." They describe the experiences as "refreshing" (Babaria et al., 2012, p. 1018). The team works differently with a non-hierarchical structure and inter-professional respect and collaboration (Babaria et al., 2012).

There is little mystery then why the practice of medicine remains so strongly gendered. The model of practice in many disciplines is male dominated, and women who participate in those groups either embrace that model and behave like their male colleagues, sometimes risking their own integrity to belong, or find other communities where they feel more comfortable and their values and skills are welcomed. This dynamic then becomes what is referred to as horizontal segregation – women restricting their career choice due to the hegemony of the model that honours more masculine qualities (Smith et al., 2018).

4. Mentorship

Mentorship is linked to success in medicine for women and men (Cruess et al., 2015; Stamm & Buddeberg-Fischer, 2011) However, it appears that women medical students are much less likely to have a mentor identified than their male colleagues (Riska, 2009; Beagan, 2000). What are the dynamics in this difference? Several authors have suggested that there is a sex difference/preference or pattern in using mentorship, that perhaps women see mentorship differently and therefore seek guidance in different ways. Others suggest that this is not so much a sociological phenomenon but a structural one whereby women are barred from the traditional forms of mentorship because of their gender. Women report that they have difficulty finding a mentor compared to their male classmates – this may be because they do not understand the "rules" of negotiating mentorship that their male colleagues understand. The other may be simply that women are seeking mentorship from women physicians who are less visible to them. This is clear from the statistics of number of women faculty and number of faculty at levels of power and influence. With women composing more than 50% of the class but less than 28% of the faculty it is simple math: there simply are not enough women faculty available, let alone visible, to mentor the women students.

Students themselves also report that their mentorship aspirations are formed by developing relationships with faculty in strategic ways to assist them in opening doors to potential career paths. Men appear to understand this strategy, with over 60% of male students reporting mentoring relationships (with either men or women as mentors) versus less than 40% of women (Rosenthal et al., 2013; Riska, 2009; Stamm & Buddeberg-Fischer, 2011). Women who report having mentors articulate strategic mentorship and go on to describe the qualities of mentorship that are important to them. Thus, having a women faculty member as a mentor is not sufficient for them, rather women students seek mentors who listen and foster a reciprocal relationship. Women appear to choose mentors who are non-hierarchical yet also connected (have power) and can actively sponsor students in career opportunities or open the doors to a community of practice (Levine et al., 2013). Other studies suggest that women want and need women as mentors and differentiate the gender difference – pointing out overall that women prefer to be mentored by women

Beyond sheer numbers, visibility, and perceived power of women faculty as mentors, it is important to appreciate the burden of mentorship for women faculty who often spend inordinate time with students who are seeking support. Women faculty simply have less time and greater obligations for student mentorship because of numbers and other responsibilities. Women faculty usually carry the burdens of far greater responsibilities for child care and eldercare than their male counterparts (Jolly et al., 2014).

Mentorship appears to be a crucial issue in the formation of professional experiences – not just from the perspective of opportunity but in the process of identity formation. Here I draw the connection between mentorship and sense of professional identity (Cruess et al., 2015; Frost & Regehr, 2013). This has a generic implication as we know that women medical students (although starting at the same place as their male colleagues) show significant decline in their self-confidence by the end of their first year of studies; by the end of medical school there is a significant difference between women and men in their readiness to take on the role of doctor (Babaria et al. 2011; Blanch et al., 2008).

Equally disturbing is the consistent evidence of the higher level of anxiety reported by women students, the impact of life stresses that women report and their self-assessment or sharing of success. These factors are significantly different for their male colleagues who themselves may overestimate their abilities. These documented differences stand in contrast to the usual evidence of academic success, where women students overall have equal or superior academic standing in their class (Blanch et al., 2008).

5. Leadership and Promotion: A Gender Imbalance in the Academy

Significant global evidence reveals the apparent mismatch between the gender balance of the student body and the faculty. Throughout Canada male faculty still considerably outnumber the female faculty, and for those schools with a greater number of women on faculty, few are full professors or department heads. In Canada, there have only been three women deans (Rochon et al., 2016; AFMC, 2016). This means that women are seen in supportive and low-influence positions by their colleagues and students. They have limited, if any, impact on important leadership and decision making in the faculty overall. This glass ceiling or vertical segregation has been articulated in the literature (Riska, 2009).

The evidence is compelling about the issues of leadership opportunities for women in medicine. Women eschew academic medicine for a variety of reasons. Some never felt at home in the academy and so never imagined an academic career; many were never encouraged or mentored to take on teaching roles; and many who joined departed because of experiences of marginalization, discounting, and the rigours of academic medicine and promotion that are not sensitive to women's life demands (raising a family, caring for aging parents) (Rochon et al., 2016). Some women are unable to consider leadership roles coupled with their other familial responsibilities. These issues have been articulated in several studies exploring the continued absence or disappearance of women in the hierarchy of medicine and academia (Pololi et al., 2012; Rochon et al., 2016).

The underlying issues are very like those experiences of women medical students. Women feel marginalized, discounted, undervalued, unworthy, unmentored, and unsupported. Some of the literature ascribes this attrition to poor advancement and salary differentials. Polili and colleagues (Pololi et al., 2012; Pololi et al., 2013) document the dissatisfactions of women faculty as unrelatedness (to other faculty and the institutional values), moral distress because of ethical challenges in the workplace, and lack of engagement (feeling invisible and isolated) as their reasons for leaving academic medicine. Faculties have been addressing this issue for greater than three decades with affirmative action programs to support women and other minority groups to remain within academia. These programs continue to be necessary despite women filling more than 50% of the undergraduate positions (Rochon et al., 2016).

There are many consequences to the absence of female leadership in the academy. For medical students, the male model of authority and leadership continues and so perpetuates the image of the male as the model of physician-ship. Students curiously come to view their women faculty differently, often harshly judging their capabilities as both physician role models and as teachers (Morgan et al., 2016). Women students lack role models and mentorship and particularly lack a vision of women having leadership, power, and influence in medical education (Bleakley, 2013). Medicine itself suffers as the qualities that women may bring to medicine through leadership is a lost resource. Why does the glass ceiling exist? Clearly, the experiences of faculty have a huge impact on the students and it is argued that this creates and perpetuates a hidden curriculum that contributes to the worrisome cynicism, loss of altruism, and erosion of the moral/ humanistic underpinnings of the practice of medicine (MacLeod, 2011).

6. Marginalization, Isolation, and Exclusion

The daily experience of women in medical training appears to be negatively affected by issues of gender. Women state that the repetitive experiences of inequity result in the feelings of not belonging or disidentification. Women find the subtle experiences, which Beagan (2005) calls "microaggressions" (p. 783), most distressing. These daily transgressions have a cumulative effect that whittles away at their self-image. Women have coping strategies that distance them either from their classmates or from themselves. Many of these are worrisome as they include self-blame, disengagement, desensitization, and resignation (Babaria et al., 2012; Phillips & Clarke, 2012). It is compelling to learn that women at the end of first year have lost self-confidence while their male colleagues report the opposite, and that by the end of their undergraduate education women students are significantly less ready to take on the role of doctor as they approach their residency (Blanch et al., 2008).

7. Hidden Curriculum

The hidden curriculum as first articulated by Haas and Shafir (1977) and then popularized by Hafferty (Hafferty & Franks, 1994; Hafferty, 1998) shapes students' experiences. It is revealed through words, behaviours, and attitudes and how medical education is delivered. Lemmp and Seale (2004) state that the impact of these processes results in loss of idealism, a ritualized professional identity, emotional neutralization and change in ethical integrity, and an unchallenged acceptance of medical hierarchy – in other words, deference and obedience.

The hidden curriculum continues to dominate the literature and reports for reform in medical education. Perpetuation of the concept of these forces as being "hidden" (AFMC, 2010) serves to support the institutional argument that what cannot be seen is impossible to modify. The literature over the past 30 years suggests that this hidden curriculum of the genderization of medicine and its impact on 50% of our students is clearly not hidden but is standing in plain view (Giles & Hill, 2015; MacLeod, 2014; Rochon et al., 2016; Smith et al., 2018).

The hidden curriculum concept is one that most likely explains the "reform without change" accusation and perhaps partly explains how the culture of medical education has remained largely unchanged (Swanson, 1989, p. 1173). Despite numerous calls for reform and many commissions of inquiry, the Lancet Commission states that professional education has not kept pace with challenges in society largely because of "fragmented, outdated and static curricula that produce ill-equipped graduates" (Frenk et al., 2010, p. 1923).

What Are the Consequences of the Barriers?

If the culture of medicine is impervious to change despite multiple pleas for reform, what are the consequences?

1. Restricted Career Choice

The evidence is pretty clear, not just in North America but globally, that women continue to "choose" medical careers in a very limited range. Women, despite composing greater than 50% of the class, disproportionately choose careers in pediatrics, family medicine, and obstetrics and gynecology.

There has been much theorizing of how and why women choose careers in these particular disciplines; overall it comes down to either a socializing influence (women choose careers they are most socialized to with characteristics associated with women – nurturing, relationships, maternal instincts) or as a consequence of barriers that restrict their choices in practical and subtle ways. Hill and Vaughn (2013, p. 548) use the concept of "paradigmatic trajectories" conceptualized by Wenger. This analysis of women's relative absence from surgical careers has been explained as the absence of a visible career path for women students which ultimately shape women's experiences of surgery as a possible career choice (Wenger, 1998).

Wenger's (1998) notion of these paradigmatic trajectories as fundamental to career paths describes the opportunities to see and experience this path as that of the community of practice. This community welcomes newcomers to the discipline. Thus, for women medical students, surgery is not a welcoming community to their legitimate participation. This is experienced through gendered experiences (women treated differently than men), a lack of role models, and a lack of or negative mentoring experiences (Hill & Vaughan, 2013; Moulton et al., 2013).

Professional identity formation (PIF) has become a major focus in the education literature. It deserves some attention in this context as it appears to be a crucial concept in understanding the development of women as physicians and in trying to understand why this culture has been slow to change. The impact of gendered experiences has had scant attention in the literature on PIF until Babaria and colleagues (2012) conducted a longitudinal qualitative study of women students in their third or clerkship year in North American medical schools. What the researchers report is a clear narrative of the gendered experiences of these students and how their professional identity adapted in response to these experiences. They argue that professional identity, like gender identity, is a dynamic process. For women medical students this includes how to enact the role of a woman doctor. This process is described as a reconciliation of identities as women and as doctors. Women report a complex and demanding navigation of what it means to be a woman doctor, often with conflicting messages about their femininity. Encouraged to demonstrate their competence, they often adopt masculine behaviours to prove their eligibility and to avoid sexually inappropriate advances by their supervisors. Yet at other times they need to embrace their feminine qualities to meet the expectations of others.

Beagan (2000) calls this a socialization process whereby women learn to adopt the prevailing male culture and neutralize their gender in their mannerisms, behaviour, and dress. This she argues is the homogenization of the class that stands in stark contrast to the calls for diversity in medicine. The forces for conformity (one-size-fits-all male model of physician) are very strong and act to nullify policies of social justice and equity that look to diversity as an answer to unmet societal needs (Razack et al., 2015).

PIF is a developmental process that all students undergo and is deeply personal. This journey is enveloped in an educational process that celebrates the need for diversity while simultaneously moving towards greater standardization in assessment. This tension between the unique medical student upon admission and the product of the education system that declares and proves competence has important consequences for PIF (Razack et al., 2015).

Societal expectations and demands that medicine train individuals who will be accountable to address gaps and deficiencies in health care has fuelled the concept of opening medical education to a wider array of students. Greater representation of students from socially disadvantaged and unrepresented populations has been a policy of most faculties of medicine in efforts to address the lack of equitable medical services in rural, inner city, and Indigenous communities. At the same time a call for increased accountability to the public by ensuring that all graduates have the competence to practise medicine has created a tension that has affected the PIF of students. Although PIF is deeply personal and emerges from the individual's values, the culture of medicine also socially constructs it. Students as emerging professionals want and need to fit in. This creates a trade-off between individual, unique contributions and the acceptance into the culture by being more alike than different. We have made the assumption in our early grasp of competency that there is a uniform way of being competent. So for those different students, accepted because of their diversity, their experience of marginalization is immense (Beagan, 2005). This difference is a great silencer for such individuals and this silence also serves to magnify the differences. This stifles and isolates many students. Added to this is the tragedy of the dominant male hegemonic models that are so pervasive and resilient that the contribution that diversity can offer is undermined (Beagan, 2005; Razack et al., 2015). So not only do women (despite their majority in the class) suffer the erosion of personal "erasure" but a similar process occurs for all students who do not conform to the white, male, middle-class model that has defined medical education for the last century (Frost & Regehr, 2013, p. 1574).

Clearly this further articulates the need for a different and central approach to PIF where diversity is welcome and homogenization of the class is minimized. How do we create a model of medical education that nurtures differences at the same time as assuring competence? Frost and Regehr (2013) explore this tension and suggest attention to a hybrid identity that is customized to each student through support and guidance. In their model students are active agents in their journey and the teacher's role is to facilitate, not stifle, and intentionally guide the process. They state that PIF should not mean erasure of one's unique identity but rather should be a personal journey for all students as they are encouraged to foster their own identity within the larger, more principally defined professional identity. They term this "identity integration" (Frost & Regehr, 2013, p. 1575). This of course would demand a fundamental change to the role of the teacher in the faculty of medicine (Cooke et al., 2010).

This complex process of PIF has been an implicit rather than explicit one in medical education and therefore subject to neglect. Added to this is the assumption that all students will undergo a similar if not exactly the same PIF, which severely underestimates the theory and science behind this crucial inauguration into the profession. Attention to this process and the unique struggles of each student will be fundamental to helping to address the persistent difficulties and marginalization of women students.

2. Coping Strategies and Mental Health Issues

What is most telling about this research is the progressive desensitization and gradual acceptance by women students of the inevitability of gendered encounters. Their assessment of the impact of these egregious behaviours encountered in the beginning of their clinical year gradually become less affronting and are minimized. When asked to explain their reaction the common refrain was one of "they are just dealing with it" or "they are just too tired to care" (Babaria et al., 2011, p. 256; Cruess et al., 2015; Frost & Regehr, 2013). This resignation and seeming acceptance of harassment even emerges in advance of their clinical years, which is when most sexual harassment and abuse occur. Women appear to accept gender discrimination and harassment as inevitable parts of the culture of medicine. They rarely report these experiences because of the well documented explanations of power dynamics of supervisory relationships, the prevalence of the events that are too numerous and "insignificant" to report, the concern about future career impact, and the lack of institutional response (MacLeod, 2011).

Similarly, in her own analysis of the puzzling perpetuation of gendered experiences and harassment Wear and colleagues (2007) wondered whether a new generation of women medical students process this experience differently. They explored the concept of the third wave of feminism whereby women students come from a generation where gender discrimination is not labelled as such, so when confronted with these challenges in medical school women's response is to "suck it up," submit, don't complain, and don't report.

They also appear to look to their female supervisors as role models who, although supportive and sympathetic to their experiences, also seem to have resigned themselves to the inevitability of these experiences through disengagement and departure from educational institutions (Rochon et al., 2016). This sadly speaks to the perpetuation of the silence around gendered experience.

The factors that shape professional identity are role models, mentorship, and the individual's experience. The Carnegie Foundation (Frenk et al., 2010) has announced that PIF should be the major focus for medical education. Cruess and colleagues (2015) are the champions of attention to PIF in Canadian medical education. They divide PIF into three domains: (1) the self or individual, (2) the relational (the impact of significant others including partners, family, and mentors), and finally, (3) the collective, which is the impact of the group that the emerging professional wants to join. They argue that understanding this developmental model is crucial for medical educators to most effectively support and nurture the student as an emerging professional. Clearly, the availability and ability of role models and mentors is central to the PIF of women students (Cruess et al., 2015).

Role models are fundamental to the PIF of professionals as students observe, practise, and imitate physicians they work with. The influence on the PIF of students, Cruess and colleagues (2015) argue, must be made explicit to nurture those qualities, values, and habits that are the foundation of their competence. This process of "making explicit" occurs through mentorship and guided reflection with a trusted other.

3. Impact on Leadership

The issue of leadership is fundamental to the exploration of the perpetuation of a hegemonic culture in medicine. As women make up at least half of the class at both the undergraduate and residency levels it was anticipated that gender equity would translate into greater opportunities for leadership among women. This pipeline approach has not been realized, with a stark absence of women in leadership roles (Rochon et al., 2016). Gender bias is still an important phenomenon in medicine and medical education with ample evidence of the limited number of women holding leadership positions.

Academic success is often predicated on the ability to conduct research and other scholarly work. Not only do women express doubts about their capabilities to meet the rigorous demands of the academic career path, but they also make career decisions based on the needs and demands of raising their families (Rochon et al., 2016; Smith et al., 2018). Academic promotion in most universities fails to recognize the different career trajectory of women and ultimately serves as a barrier to women pursuing academic roles. This burden is also cited as the reason many women refuse possible leadership positions (Rochon et al., 2016).

Women appear to be excluded from academy through gender bias in both publication and granting agencies (Rochon et al., 2016; Jagsi et al., 2006; "*Nature*'s Sexism," 2012). In a serious challenge to equity in publication, Dickersin and colleagues (1998) investigated the gender based publication bias in four major medical journals. These studies revealed significant gender imbalance in academic publication with almost 90% of editors, 73% of reviewers, and 70% of authors being male. Budden et al. (2008) pursued this question in comparing journals who used a double-blind process in their editorial process. It appears that this process increases the number of women authors. The journal *Nature* conducted its own internal audit in 2012 after being challenged about the number of women writers in the journal. To its credit it published this review, titled "*Nature*'s Sexism" (2012). It discovered that the gender bias for the journal is significant and clearly not representative of the number of women academics ("*Nature*'s Sexism," 2012). This led to a declaration that it will encourage an editorial policy decision to consider "who are the five women I could ask?" about commissioned articles. It is clear through this brief analysis of gender bias in publication that it is real and that there may be effective strategies to mitigate this bias through double-blind reviews and affirmative action on the part of editors.

If leadership and publication bias require affirmative action to level the playing field, then earlier intervention in the career trajectory of women seems prudent. Wayne and colleagues (2010) explored the gender differences in leadership among first-year medical students learning in small groups. Strikingly it revealed that disproportionately fewer women than men became group leaders even in a course that had women leaders as faculty. Interestingly, this study also included a simple intervention with half the class that appeared to significantly increase the number of women students stepping into leadership roles. The faculty simply instructed all the students to consider volunteering to be leaders of the group as it was an important experience for everyone to have and that this was a low-risk, safe environment.

The barriers to women's full participation in medicine then must be addressed with attention to a philosophy of equity and inclusiveness by challenges to the dominant cultural traditions that exclude women and ultimately with affirmative action that purposefully addresses the issues that serve as barriers to women's full participation in medicine.

Special Skills and Attributes That Women Bring to Medicine

Not only is this an issue of equity for women in medicine and society in general, but perhaps more compelling are the contributions to the much-needed transformation of medicine that women can bring to medicine (Frenk et al., 2010; AFMC, 2010).

Social accountability. Current issues in health care reform have focused on the social accountability mandate of medical schools (AFMC, 2010). In a recent study of medical graduates in Canada, Smith and colleagues (2018) have uncovered interesting differences between men and women and their commitment to issues of social justice and accountability in their career considerations. Women as undergraduate applicants to medicine articulate issues of social accountability more frequently, and this may have impact on the interview process and acceptance of a larger number of women (W. Parsons, assistant dean of admissions, Memorial University, personal communication, 2017; Steering Committee on Social Accountability of Medical Schools, 2001). Women medical students do more often select family medicine as a career choice, and this may in part reflect a commitment to the underserved in primary care.

Clinical skills and health outcomes. Women appear to have superior clinical outcomes in hospital-based medicine. A recent study published in *JAMA* suggests that patients who had women attending physicians were more likely to survive (Tsugawa et al., 2017). The authors comment on a variety of explanatory models to account for this difference, including women's attention to evidence-based medicine; their overall superior clinical performance in standardized clinical skills testing; and their patient-centredness, which results in more time per patient, fewer investigations, and increased patient satisfaction (Roter & Hall, 2004, p. 53; Stewart et al., 2003).

Communication skills. Communication skills have long been recognized as an attribute of women physicians. Numerous studies acknowledge the impact of communication skills in patient health outcomes, and others have described women's strengths in communication (Kurtz et al., 1994; Roter & Hall, 2004; Stewart, 1995; Stewart & Gilbert, 2005). This *JAMA* study now clearly makes linkages between communication style and patient survival in the hospital setting.

Linked clearly with communication skills is the patient-centred approach that has a positive impact on patient satisfaction, improves adherence to medical advice, and reduces investigations, all of which improve health care outcomes and reduce health care costs. Women physicians are more likely to be patient centred in their practice. Medicine and health care in general gain from this approach. (Stewart & Gilbert, 2005, p. 53)

Inter-professional approaches. Inter-professional approaches to health care have been advocated as the way to improve quality of health and patient safety. Women physicians are more likely to work inter-professionally and are vital role models for future physicians on how to work effectively in the inter-professional environment (Carr et al., 2009).

Call to Action

Affirmative Action

The need for affirmative action is clear (Sklar, 2016) and should be targeted at the barriers that have been identified. First, a zero-tolerance policy about sexual harassment and sexual abuse is vital to ensure that women are safe in their learning environment. As in other complex organizations, this will require support through university and medical school structures to ultimately eradicate (National Defence and the Canadian Armed Forces, 2017).

Women are a marginalized group (despite their proportional numbers) and so can bring focus to the whole culture of medicine and its dominant values and hidden curriculum, which marginalize many others. At a time when health care reforms call for diversity, medicine at its core fosters conformity, nullifying the movement towards diversification and inclusiveness in admissions policies. The need to focus on the individual student and his or her unique contribution to their class and the future of health care requires serious attention to the professional identity formation of future physicians (MacLeod & Frank, 2013).

Leadership by (and for) women is a huge challenge and must be addressed through affirmative action. Many barriers exist to women's full participation in leadership roles. This is not just an issue in medicine. Structural changes to medicine, academic promotion, and mentorship are required to ensure that women consider and are supported in accepting and pursuing leadership. It is only when women have proportional representation in the leadership of faculties, departments, organizations, and health care systems that they will be enabled to effectively contribute to the reformation of medical education and health care delivery overall.

In the words of the editor of *Academic Medicine*: "We do not need more articles [or chapters] that describe the problems of women in medicine. There are now well recognized. What we need is the courage and commitment to solve the problems" (Sklar, 2016).

It is time to see and hear the voices of women in medicine.

ACKNOWLEDGMENT

I would like to thank and acknowledge three significant contributors to this chapter: Wendy Graham (Memorial University), Allyn Walsh (McMaster University), and Bob Miller (Northern Ontario School of Medicine).

REFERENCES

Acker, J. (1990). Hierarchies, jobs, bodies: A theory of gendered organizations.*Gender and Society*, *4*(2), 139–58.

Alers, M., van Leerdam, L., Dielissen, P., & Lagro-Janssen, A. (2014, Jun). Gendered specialities during medical education: A literature review. *Perspectives on Medical Education*, *3*(3), 163–78. https://doi.org/10.1007/s40037-014-0132-1 Medline:24980516

Association of Faculties of Medicine of Canada. (2010). *The future of medical education in Canada (FMEC): A collective vison for MD education*. Ottawa: Author.

Association of Faculties of Medicine of Canada. (2016). 2015 Canadian medical education statistics. Retrieved from https://www.afmc.ca/publications/canadian-medical-education-statistics-cmes/archives

Babaria, P., Abedin, S., Berg, D., & Nunez-Smith, M. (2012, Apr). "I'm too used to it": A longitudinal qualitative study of third year female medical students' experiences of gendered encounters in medical education. *Social Science & Medicine (1982)*, *74*(7), 1013–20. https://doi.org/10.1016/j.socscimed.2011.11.043 Medline:22341202

Babaria, P., Bernheim, S., & Nunez-Smith, M. (2011, Mar). Gender and the pre-clinical experiences of female medical students: A taxonomy. *Medical Education*, *45*(3), 249–60. https://doi.org/10.1111/j.1365-2923.2010.03856.x Medline:21299600

Beagan, B.L. (2000, Oct). Neutralizing differences: Producing neutral doctors for (almost) neutral patients. *Social Science & Medicine (1982)*, *51*(8), 1253–65. https://doi.org/10.1016/S0277-9536(00)00043-5 Medline:11037215

Beagan, B.L. (2005, Aug). Everyday classism in medical school: Experiencing marginality and resistance. *Medical Education*, *39*(8), 777–84. https://doi.org/10.1111/j.1365-2929.2005.02225.x Medline:16048620

Blanch, D.C., Hall, J.A., Roter, D.L., & Frankel, R.M. (2008, Sep). Medical student gender and issues of confidence. *Patient Education and Counseling*, *72*(3), 374–81. https://doi.org/10.1016/j.pec.2008.05.021 Medline:18656322

Bleakley, A. (2013). Gender matters in medical education. *Medical Education*, *47*, 59–70. https://doi.org/10.1111/j.1365-2923.2012.04351.x

British Medical Journal. (2016). This is what we look like. Retrieved from http://careers.bmj.com/careers/advice/view-article.html?id=20022883

Budden, A.E., Tregenza, T., Aarssen, L.W., Koricheva, J., Leimu, R., & Lortie, C.J. (2008, Jan). Double-blind review favours increased representation of female authors. *Trends in Ecology & Evolution*, *23*(1), 4–6. https://doi.org/10.1016/j.tree.2007.07.008 Medline:17963996

Carr, P.L., Pololi, L., Knight, S., & Conrad, P. (2009, Oct). Collaboration in academic medicine: reflections on gender and advancement. *Academic Medicine: Journal of the Association of American Medical Colleges*, *84*(10), 1447–53. https://doi.org/10.1097/ACM.0b013e3181b6ac27 Medline:19881441

Cheng, L.-F., & Yang, H.-C. (2015, Mar). Learning about gender on campus: An analysis of the hidden curriculum for medical students. *Medical Education*, *49*(3), 321–31. https://doi.org/10.1111/medu.12628 Medline:25693991

Cooke, M., Irby, D., O'Brien, B., & Shuhan, L. (2010). *Educating physicians: A call for reform of medical school and residency*. Hoboken, NJ: Jossey-Bass.

Cruess, R.L., Cruess, S.R., Boudreau, D., Snell, L., & Steinert, Y. (2015). A schematic representation of the professional identity formation and socialization of medical students and residents: A guide for medical

educators. *Academic Medicine: Journal of the Association of American Medical Colleges, 90*(6), 1–8.
Dickersin, K., Fredman, L., Flegal, K.M., Scott, J.D., & Crawley, B. (1998, Jul 15). Is there a sex bias in choosing editors? Epidemiology journals as an example. *JAMA, 280*(3), 260–4. https://doi.org/10.1001/jama.280.3.260 Medline:9676675
Dolishny, V.N., & Noelle, V. (2012). "Proving yourself" in the Canadian medical profession: Gender and the experiences of foreign-trained doctors in medical practices. University of Western Ontario-Electronic thesis and dissertation repository. Paper 880.
Frost, H.D., & Regehr, G. (2013, Oct). "I AM a doctor": Negotiating the discourses of standardization and diversity in professional identity construction. *Academic Medicine: Journal of the Association of American Medical Colleges, 88*(10), 1570–7. https://doi.org/10.1097/ACM.0b013e3182a34b05 Medline:23969361
Frenk, J., Chen, L., Bhutta, Z.A., Cohen, J., Crisp, N., Evans, T., …, & Zurayk, H. (2010, Dec 4). Health professionals for a new century: Transforming education to strengthen health systems in an interdependent world. *Lancet, 376*(9756), 1923–58. https://doi.org/10.1016/S0140-6736(10)61854-5 Medline:21112623
Giles, J.A., & Hill, E.J.R. (2015, Mar). Examining our hidden curricula: Powerful, visible, gendered and discriminatory. *Medical Education, 49*(3), 244–6. https://doi.org/10.1111/medu.12664 Medline:25693983
Haas, J., & Shaffir, W. (1977). The professionalization of medical students: Developing competence and a cloak of confidence. *Symbolic Interaction, 1*(1), 71–88. https://doi.org/10.1525/si.1977.1.1.71
Hafferty, F.W., & Franks, R. (1994, Nov). The hidden curriculum, ethics teaching, and the structure of medical education. *Academic Medicine: Journal of the Association of American Medical Colleges, 69*(11), 861–71. https://doi.org/10.1097/00001888-199411000-00001 Medline:7945681
Hafferty, F.W. (1998, Apr). Beyond curriculum reform: Confronting medicine's hidden curriculum. *Academic Medicine: Journal of the Association of American Medical Colleges, 73*(4), 403–7. https://doi.org/10.1097/00001888-199804000-00013 Medline:9580717
Hill, E., Bowman, K., Stalmeijer, R., & Hart, J. (2014, Sep). You've got to know the rules to play the game: How medical students negotiate the hidden curriculum of surgical careers. *Medical Education, 48*(9), 884–94. https://doi.org/10.1111/medu.12488 Medline:25113115
Hill, E.J., & Giles, J.A. (2014, Jun). Career decisions and gender: The illusion of choice? *Perspectives on Medical Education, 3*(3), 151–4. https://doi.org/10.1007/s40037-014-0128-x Medline:24957796

Hill, E., & Vaughan, S. (2013, Jun). The only girl in the room: How paradigmatic trajectories deter female students from surgical careers. *Medical Education, 47*(6), 547–56. https://doi.org/10.1111/medu.12134 Medline:23662871

Jagsi, R., Guancial, E.A., Worobey, C.C., Henault, L.E., Chang, Y., Starr, R., …, & Hylek, E.M. (2006, Jul 20). The "gender gap" in authorship of academic medical literature: A 35-year perspective. *The New England Journal of Medicine, 355*(3), 281–7. https://doi.org/10.1056/NEJMsa053910 Medline:16855268

Jolly, S., Griffith, K.A., DeCastro, R., Stewart, A., Ubel, P., & Jagsi, R. (2014, Mar 4). Gender differences in time spent on parenting and domestic responsibilities by high-achieving young physician-researchers. *Annals of Internal Medicine, 160*(5), 344–53. https://doi.org/10.7326/M13-0974 Medline:24737273

Kurtz, S.M., Silverman, J.D., & Draper, J. (1994). *Teaching and learning communication skills in medicine*. Oxford, England: Radcliffe Medical Press.

Lempp, H., & Seale, C. (2004, Oct 2). The hidden curriculum in undergraduate medical education: Qualitative study of medical students' perceptions of teaching. *BMJ (Clinical Research Ed.), 329*(7469), 770–3. https://doi.org/10.1136/bmj.329.7469.770 Medline:15459051

Levine, R.B., Mechaber, H.F., Reddy, S.T., Cayea, D., & Harrison, R.A. (2013, Apr). "A good career choice for women": Female medical students' mentoring experiences: a multi-institutional qualitative study. *Academic Medicine: Journal of the Association of American Medical Colleges, 88*(4), 527–34. https://doi.org/10.1097/ACM.0b013e31828578bb Medline:23425983

Lockwood, P., & Kunda, Z. (1997). Superstars and Me: Predicting the impact of role models on the self. *Journal of Personality and Social Psychology, 73*(1), 91–103. https://doi.org/10.1037/0022-3514.73.1.91

MacLeod, A. (2011, Aug). Caring, competence and professional identities in medical education. *Advances in Health Sciences Education: Theory and Practice, 16*(3), 375–94. https://doi.org/10.1007/s10459-010-9269-9 Medline:21188513

MacLeod, A. (2014, Jun). The hidden curriculum: Is it time to re-consider the concept? *Medical Teacher, 36*(6), 539–40. https://doi.org/10.3109/0142159X.2014.907876 Medline:24787524

MacLeod, A., & Frank, B. (2013, Jan). Feminist pedagogy and medical education: Why not now? *Medical Education, 47*(1), 11–14. https://doi.org/10.1111/medu.12095 Medline:23278818

Morgan, H., Purkiss, J.A., Porter, A.C., Lypson, M.L., Santen, S.A., Christner, J.G., . . . Hammoud, M.M. (2016). Student evaluation of faculty physicians:

Gender differences in teaching evaluations. *Journal of Women's Health, 25*(5), 453–6. https://doi.org/10.1089/jwh.2015.5475

Moulton, C.A., Seemann, N., & Webster, F. (2013, Jun). It's all about gender, or is it? *Medical Education, 47*(6), 538–40. https://doi.org/10.1111/medu.12196 Medline:23662867

National Defence and the Canadian Armed Forces. (2017). *Internal review of workplace policies, programs and leadership engagement.* Retrieved from http://www.forces.gc.ca/en/caf-community-support-services/internal-review.page

Nature's sexism. (2012). *Nature, 491*(7425), 495. https://doi.org/10.1038/491495a

Phillips, C.B. (2009, Sep). Student portfolios and the hidden curriculum on gender: mapping exclusion. *Medical Education, 43*(9), 847–53. https://doi.org/10.1111/j.1365-2923.2009.03403.x Medline:19709009

Phillips, S., & Clarke, M. (2012). More than an education: The hidden curriculum, professional attitudes, and career choice. *Medical Education, 46*(9), 887–93. https://doi.org/10.1111/j.1365-2923.2012.04316.x

Pololi, L.H., Civian, J.T., Brennan, R.T., Dottolo, A.L., & Krupat, E. (2013). Experiencing the culture of academic medicine: Gender matters, a national study. *Journal of General Internal Medicine, 28*(2), 201–7. Medline:22936291

Pololi, L.H., Krupat, E., Civian, J.T., Ash, A.S., & Brennan, R.T. (2012, Jul). Why are a quarter of faculty considering leaving academic medicine? A study of their perceptions of institutional culture and intentions to leave at 26 representative U.S. medical schools. *Academic Medicine: Journal of the Association of American Medical Colleges, 87*(7), 859–69. https://doi.org/10.1097/ACM.0b013e3182582b18 Medline:22622213

Razack, S., Hodges, B., Steinert, Y., & Maguire, M. (2015, Jan). Seeking inclusion in an exclusive process: Discourses of medical school student selection. *Medical Education, 49*(1), 36–47. https://doi.org/10.1111/medu.12547 Medline:25545572

Riska, E. (2009). Gender and medical education. In C. Brosnan & B.S. Turner (Eds.), *Handbook of the sociology of medical education* (pp. 89–105). London: Routledge.

Rochon, P.A., Davidoff, F., & Levinson, W. (2016, Aug). Women in academic medicine leadership: Has anything changed in 25 years? *Academic Medicine: Journal of the Association of American Medical Colleges, 91*(8), 1053–6. https://doi.org/10.1097/ACM.0000000000001281 Medline:27306972

Rosenthal, L., Levy, S.R., London, B., Lobel, M., & Bazile, C. (2013, Apr). In pursuit of the MD: The impact of role models, identity compatibility, and belonging among undergraduate women. *Sex Roles, 68*(7–8), 464–73. https://doi.org/10.1007/s11199-012-0257-9 Medline:24497671

Roter, D.L., & Hall, J.A. (2004). Physician gender and patient-centered communication: A critical review of empirical research. *Annual Review of Public Health, 25*(1), 497–519. https://doi.org/10.1146/annurev.publhealth.25.101802.123134 Medline:15015932

Sklar, D.P. (2016, Aug). Women in medicine: Enormous progress, stubborn challenges. *Academic Medicine: Journal of the Association of American Medical Colleges, 91*(8), 1033–5. https://doi.org/10.1097/ACM.0000000000001259 Medline:27465080

Smith, V., Bethune, C., & Hurley, K.F. (2018, Jan-Mar). Examining medical student specialty choice through a gender lens: An orientational qualitative study. *Teaching and Learning in Medicine, 30*(1), 33–44.

Stamm, M., & Buddeberg-Fischer, B. (2011, May). The impact of mentoring during postgraduate training on doctors' career success. *Medical Education, 45*(5), 488–96. https://doi.org/10.1111/j.1365-2923.2010.03857.x Medline:21486324

Steering Committee on Social Accountability of Medical Schools. (2001). Social accountability: A vision for Canadian medical schools. Ottawa: Minister of Public Works and Government Services Canada.

Stewart, M., & Gilbert, B. (2005). Reflections on the doctor-patient relationship: From evidence and experience. *British Journal of General Practice, 55*(519), 793–801.

Stewart, M.A. (1995, May 1). Effective physician-patient communication and health outcomes: a review. *CMAJ, 152*(9), 1423–1433. Medline:7728691

Stewart, M., Brown, J.B., Weston, W.W., McWhinney, I.R., McWilliam, C.L., & Freeman, T.R. (2003). *Patient-centred medicine*. Oxford, England: Radcliffe.

Swanson, A. (1989). Medical education reform without change. *Mayo Clinical Proceedings, 64*, 1173–4.

Tsugawa, Y., Jena, A.B., Figueroa, J.F., Orav, E.J., Blumenthal, D.M., & Jha, A.K. (2017, Feb 1). Comparison of hospital mortality and readmission rates for medicare patients treated by male vs female physicians. *JAMA Internal Medicine, 177*(2), 206–13. https://doi.org/10.1001/jamainternmed.2016.7875 Medline:27992617

Wayne, N.L., Vermillion, M., & Uijtdehaage, S. (2010, Aug). Gender differences in leadership amongst first-year medical students in the small-group setting. *Academic Medicine: Journal of the Association of American Medical Colleges, 85*(8), 1276–81. https://doi.org/10.1097/ACM.0b013e3181e5f2ce Medline:20671452

Wear, D., Aultman, J.M., & Borges, N.J. (2007, Winter). Retheorizing sexual harassment in medical education: Women students' perceptions at five U.S.

medical schools. *Teaching and Learning in Medicine, 19*(1), 20–9. https://doi.org/10.1080/10401330709336619 Medline:17330995

Wenger, E. (1998). *Communities of practice. Learning, meaning and identity.* Cambridge: Cambridge University Press. https://doi.org/10.1017/CBO9780511803932

6 Female International Medical Graduates in Canada

INGE SCHABORT

This chapter is dedicated to the thousands of IMGs in Canada.

I felt small and insignificant. I felt like a number. I found the role of unemployed immigrant much more difficult than I could have imagined. I was lonely, frustrated and angry. I felt locked out of society. I felt I was contributing nothing. Although I had very recently been a competent autonomous professional, I began to doubt the value of my experience, of my education, and my abilities.

– Female IMG trying to enter the Canadian medical system (Association of Faculties of Medicine of Canada, 2006)

You felt dehumanized, in a sense, as if you had lost something that you had already achieved. That [your profession] had been taken away from you.

– IMG describing feelings of loss when immigrating to Canada (Wong & Lohfeld, 2008, p. 56)

In this chapter my objective as a female international medical graduate (IMG) is to provide a window into the world of female IMGs and their perspectives and experiences entering the Canadian system, training in the Canadian health care system, and practising in the Canadian system. In preparing for this paper, I surveyed female IMGs from across the country to get first-hand accounts of their experiences. The process of anonymous fluid surveys was reviewed with the McMaster Hamilton Integrated Research Ethics Board and because the email contributions to the fluid survey were anonymous, informed, and voluntary, a reply to the fluid survey implied informed consent. Two researchers, AR and DE, individually conducted a content analysis whereby they compared women's narratives with predominant themes described in the literature and organized those themes to show how female IMG narratives align with them. The survey reflects a growing body of perceptions among women IMG students and physicians. Where possible, I will supplement the discussion with narratives that have been written by female IMGs about their experiences in the Canadian medical environment.

Definition of International Medical Graduate

In the Canadian medical education context, an IMG is a student or graduate of a non-North American accredited medical school. This definition has no reference to citizenship or legal status in Canada. There are three distinct types of IMGs in the Canadian postgraduate system:

1. Immigrant IMG physicians
2. Canadians who left Canada to attend medical school abroad, also called Canadians studying abroad (CSAs)
3. Visa physicians who obtain a visa for postgraduate training in Canada and return to their home country after completion

All these groups ultimately seek licensure in Canada. Some immigrant IMGs may have the qualifications to be considered for entry to practise; however, many attempt to qualify for entry through postgraduate training programs. CSAs generally have no previous postgraduate training. Both groups must apply to the Canadian Resident Matching Service (CaRMS) for postgraduate training (Szafran et al., 2005). Visa trainees are physicians whose postgraduate education is sponsored by their country of origin. They are selected directly into the postgraduate system by the medical schools and do not compete with either the CSA or the immigrant IMG physician for positions in Canada through CaRMS. All three categories of IMGs compete for limited training resources. Some immigrant IMGs have the qualifications to be considered for entry to practise without completing further postgraduate training (Walsh et al., 2011).

Historical Background about IMGs in Canada

The First Female IMG in Canada

Historically, women have overcome numerous barriers in order to gain entrance into the medical profession. Women were not allowed to attend medical school in the United States or Canada until the mid and late 1800s, respectively.

The first female IMG to practise medicine in Canada was most likely Dr James Barry. The lengths to which this physician went to practise medicine is instructive for IMGs.

James Miranda Stuart Barry, army physician and surgeon (born c 1795 in England; died 1865 at London, England) was born Margaret Ann Bulkley in County Cork in 1795. Her mother was the sister of *James Barry*, a renowned artist and member of the Royal Academy in London. Her father was a grocer. Margaret was a bright child who wanted to become a physician, but at the time women were barred from medical school ("Barry, James Miranda Stuart," 2008; Brandon, 2018; du Preez, 2008, 2012; Kubba, 2001; Leitch, 2001; Nightingale, n.d.).

Margaret's uncle James Barry had influential friends, one of whom was General Francesca *Miranda* from Venezuela. Another friend, David *Stuart* Erskine, 11th Earl of Buchan, was an avid supporter of education of women. It is thought that General Miranda and Erskine were part of a group who planned for Margaret to enter medical school disguised as a man. After qualifying, she would be free to go to Venezuela to practise as a female physician. Thus, James Miranda Stuart Barry arrived at Edinburgh University where he entered the school of medicine in 1809 at the age of 14. The plan to go to Venezuela faltered when General Miranda was imprisoned by the Spanish and ended with his death in prison in 1816.

After graduating in medicine, Barry joined the British Army. Serving in South Africa, the Caribbean, Crimea, Corfu, Malta, Jamaica, Canada and other parts of the world, Barry gained a reputation as an outstanding surgeon. As inspector-general of military hospitals, Barry spent some months in the Crimea, studying the appalling hospital death rates in Florence Nightingale's (n.d.) Scutari hospital. Barry's visit to Crimea led to a radical reform of battlefield medicine. Barry performed the first caesarian section in Africa in which both mother and baby survived. The grateful parents named their child James Barry Munnik Hertzog in his honour. (Hertzog later became prime minister of South Africa from 1924 to 1939). Dr Barry advocated for good hygiene in hospitals, and Barry's radical treatment for leprosy and tropical diseases transformed the hospitals in which these diseases were treated.

In 1857 Barry was posted to Canada as inspector general of military hospitals, the army's senior doctor in Canada. Small and slim, and with no hair on his face, he was considered eccentric. Barry wore three-inch inserts in his shoes to increase his height from five feet and wore oversized clothing. Barry was known to have fought duels in defence of his honour. The *Canadian Encyclopedia* ("Barry, James," 2008) states Barry liked to drive around Montreal in a bright red sleigh, accompanied by a small white dog (called Psyche) and a manservant. Barry's long-kept secret was discovered when he died of dysentery and was laid out for burial in 1865. Barry is buried in Kensal Green Cemetery in London. His gravestone is marked "Dr James Barry Inspector General of Hospitals, died 26 July 1865, Aged 70 years."

IMGs in Canada Since

IMGs have played a longstanding role in providing care to Canadians. In 2010, 16,728 IMGs were licensed to practise in Canada (Canadian Institute for Health Information, 2010). This represents 24.0% of the 69,699 active physicians in that year. The proportion of IMGs in the physician workforce varies significantly across jurisdictions, ranging from 11.0% in Quebec to 47.1% in Saskatchewan. IMGs constitute approximately 31% of the doctor workforce in the United Kingdom and 25% in the United States (Huijskens et al., 2010). Over the last 10 years, the number of IMGs seeking fellowship training has increased by as much as 168%, with IMG fellows accounting for 70% of all fellows in some institutions (Sockalingam et al., 2014).

According to the CAPER IMG report in 2008 (Canadian Post-MD Education Registry, 2013), over 830 IMGs obtained a license to practise in Canada. Of these, 128 had received some postgraduate training in Canada, while 698 had gone directly to some form of licensure. In 2009, 1076 (or 40%) of new entries to practise across Canada were IMGs, with 375 of that total having received some postgraduate training in Canada. During that same period, 1765 Canadian-trained physicians entered practice. As of March 2010, there were 1916 IMGs in postgraduate training in Canada (excluding visa trainees). In 2010, approximately 450 first-year postgraduate positions across Canada were available for IMGs to enter postgraduate training. According to CAPER (Canadian Post-MD Education Registry, 2013), there were 617 IMGs in R-1 positions in 2010; the difference was American graduates (less than 30) and visa trainees.

The proportion of medical trainees who are women in Canada has increased in the past few decades. From 2004–05 to 2013–14 the proportion of female first-year post-MD trainees fluctuated between 56%

and 60%. In 2013–14, 63% of physicians exiting family medicine training programs were female, and 52% of those exiting medical, surgical, and laboratory programs were women (Canadian Post-MD Education Registry, 2013). Among first year post MD-trainees, IMGs increased in number and as a proportion of all first year trainees up until 2009–10. However, the number and proportion of IMGs dropped from 467 (17%) in 2009–10 to 426 (15%) in 2010–11. In 2013–14, 486 IMGs accounted for 16% of all first-year post-MD trainees (Canadian Post-MD Education Registry, 2013).

Recent Statistics: Licences Issued to Female IMGs

Female IMGs licensed from 2007 to 2011 receiving full licences by province were 132 in British Columbia (of the 132, female IMGs received 35.9% of total full licenses issued to IMGs); Alberta, 32.5%; Saskatchewan, 35.9%; Ontario, 37.3%; New Brunswick, 22.8%; and Nova Scotia, 27.3%. Gender categorization of licenses by IMG category is not available for all provinces (Canadian Post-MD Education Registry, 2012). Female IMGs receiving "all other categories of licenses" from 2007 and 2011 by province were 280 in BC (female IMGs received 34.6% of total other categories licenses issued to IMGs); Alberta, 32.5%; Saskatchewan, 29.8%; Ontario, 33.2%; New Brunswick, 22.1%; and Nova Scotia, 25.3%. Gender categorization of licenses by IMG category is not available for all provinces (Canadian Post-MD Education Registry, 2012).

The Official Process for IMGs to Recertify

The process of entering the medical system for IMGs has been described by IMGs as stressful, confusing, and non-transparent. Looking at the process from the historical perspective of creating a national strategy to enhance the integration of IMGs reveals a complex series of events:

I came to Canada in 2001 filled with hopes that I will be practicing medicine sooner than later because I knew about the deficiency of physicians in Canada. I was very optimistic and began to inquire about what I should do, wrote an exam after an exam including the TOEFL exam although I was taught in English. I decided to surround myself with people on the same boat as me; we created groups to help and encourage each other during our exam preparation. The struggle was always there because whenever we took a step forward and succeeded, we faced another harder step. Many time we asked ourselves, what do we really need to do to get there? This was the hardest question, because there were no clear requirements to get into a residency program. Some IMGs were much luckier than others; as those with the minimal qualifications were able to receive a spot into different programs. On the other hand, those with higher qualifications did not!

– Narrative of female IMG about trying to enter the medical system in Canada (fluidsurvey)

The contribution and role of IMGs have become apparent in numerous systematic evaluations of the Canadian health care system. The Kirby (2002) report on the state of the health care system in Canada emphasized the need for a national strategy to enhance the integration of IMGs. Soon after, the Romanow Commission (2002) report *Building on Values: The Future of Health Care in Canada* and the Human Health Resources (HHR) planning strategy considered the processes IMGs have to undertake to enter into the physician workforce. Aligned with the call for collaborative HHR planning, the 2003 First Ministers' Accord on Health Care Renewal (Health Canada, 2003) supported evidence-based initiatives to develop an information base to facilitate the integration of IMGs and increase the recruitment and retention of the health workforce (Health Canada, 2004).

The creation of the Canadian Task Force on Licensure of IMGs in 2002 was a key step in addressing the issues faced by IMGs in Canada. Recognizing their importance in Canada's health care delivery system, the taskforce made six recommendations to address IMG barriers to licensure and practice (Federal/Provincial/Territorial Advisory Committee on Health Delivery and Human Resources, 2004):

1. Increase the capacity to assess and prepare IMGs for licensure.
2. Work towards standardization of licensure.
3. Expand or develop supports/programs to assist IMGs with the licensure process and requirements in Canada.
4. Develop orientation programs to support faculty and physicians working with IMGs.
5. Develop capacity to track and recruit IMGs.
6. Develop a national research agenda, including evaluation of the IMG strategy.

Responding to recommendation 5, CAPER began work on the National IMG Database in 2005. The effort has been supported by the

Association of Faculties of Medicine of Canada (AFMC) and the Foreign Credentials Recognition Division of Human Resources and Skills Development Canada.

Phase I of the National IMG Database project focused on building a data-sharing partnership among all agencies that IMGs encounter as they progress towards medical licensure within Canada. The initial project work also involved defining sector-specific data sets to support research and statistical reporting on the flow of IMGs. By the end of phase I, in May 2009, IMG assessment centres, national medical examination and certification bodies, postgraduate medical education training programs, and medical regulatory authorities were all contributing annual data files to the National IMG Database. The first annual National IMG Database Report was published in 2009. The report provided a new and comprehensive statistical overview of the number of IMGs passing Canada's assessment, training, examination, certification and licensing processes. Phase II of the National IMG Database started in November 2009 as part of the IMGs in Canada Project, again led by CAPER. The IMGs in Canada Project was also developed to push towards a collaborative analytical agenda that supports the information and dissemination needs of data providers, planners, decision makers, and other stakeholders.

Not surprisingly, IMGs have found the IMG entry process in Canada extremely confusing. There are currently more than 60 different combinations of qualifications that entitle individuals to be licensed as physicians in various Canadian jurisdictions. Developments like Chapter 7 of the Agreement on Internal Trade and the Pan-Canadian Framework for the Assessment and Recognition of Foreign Qualifications are driving change within the regulatory environment. Most recently, the Federation of Medical Regulatory Authorities of Canada and the Medical Council of Canada (MCC) are developing a national process of application for medical registration in Canada. The MCC has also partnered with Canada's IMG assessment centres and other stakeholder organizations on the National Assessment Collaboration, which will bring greater standardization to IMG assessment for entry to postgraduate medical education. In addition to national projects, the regulatory environment has been incrementally transformed by provincial initiatives such as the Québec-France Mutual Recognition Arrangement and Ontario's simplified registration for qualified international medical doctors (Broten, 2008).

Future studies of the IMGs in Canada Project will hopefully tell us if system changes benefit IMGs and the patients who require their care.

Canadians Studying Abroad

To complicate matters further, growing numbers of Canadians have recently left Canada to study medicine abroad. Over the past several years there has been an increasing interest in Canada in learning more about CSAs and the schools where they study. A formal survey was done among CSAs by CaRMS, who released a comprehensive report on CSAs in 2010 (Canadian Resident Matching Service [CaRMS], 2010b). The report included the demographics and individual educational experiences of these Canadians who leave to train in medicine abroad, as well as the barriers that impeded these students from returning home. This information was crucial in planning how to effectively integrate these returning CSAs into our Canadian health human resources planning. The study estimated that in 2010 there were approximately 3500 Canadian students enrolled in medical schools abroad, many of them sharing the desire to return home to Canada to practise medicine.

CSAs represent a significant group of potential physicians who could supplement our physician workforce; however, governments, policymakers, and medical education faculty lack detailed information about this group of students about the current CSA numbers and details. Relevant information from the CaRMS (2010b) report included that the majority of CSAs (46.3%) were in Caribbean schools. The 2010 CSA cohort demographics (CaRMS, 2010a) concluded that overall there was a higher percentage of male students (52.5%) enrolled in international medical schools than males in Canadian medical schools (41.8%) (Association of Faculties of Medicine of Canada, [AFMC], 2009). Irish medical schools were the exception, with 57.0% female students, which is similar in composition to Canadian medical schools, which average 58.2% female students (AFMC, 2009).

Overall, CSAs are older than students in Canadian medical schools: 73.9% of CSAs are 26 to 30 years old while only 46.4% of Canadian medical graduates (CMGs) are the same age (Canadian Resident Matching Service, 2010a). A higher percentage of CSAs are single (83.1%) compared to students studying medicine in Canada (61.6%) (Canadian Resident Matching Service, 2010a).

An interesting finding was that CSAs were more often children of physicians, with 21.0% reporting one or more of their parents as medical doctors compared to 15.6% of CMGs (Collier, 2010). CSAs whose parents were physicians were more likely to attend medical school in Ireland, and the majority of CSAs came from British Columbia and Ontario. One reason that CSAs were older than Canadian graduates may be that despite the fact that some CSAs were entering medical school directly from high school (5.9% of CSAs), more CSAs had advanced degrees than students in Canada, with 13.1% of CSAs reporting master's degrees, while 9.8% of CMGs reported the same level of education (AFMC, 2009). CSAs applied to Canadian medical schools an average of 1.76 times while CMGs applied 2.59 times before being accepted (AFMC, 2009). Also of note was that 26.7% of CSAs had never applied to a Canadian medical school. The most frequently reported reason for choosing an international medical school was that students felt they would be unable to secure a place in a Canadian school.

While most CSAs (over 90%) reported wanting to return to Canada for postgraduate training, they report frustration with the perceived barriers to pursuing postgraduate education in Canada. These barriers include the choice of discipline, the return of service, and the high competition for positions. The CaRMS (2010b) report also states that while Canada has a ubiquitous shortage of family physicians, particularly in rural communities, only 21% of CSAs on the CaRMS survey chose a career in family medicine. However, they report having very few, if any, opportunities to complete postgraduate training in the country where they are studying medicine. None of the for-profit schools in the Caribbean have postgraduate training opportunities, and the schools that recruit Canadian students in Ireland, Poland, other European countries, and Australia have little or no postgraduate opportunities available for international students. Admission data provided by the schools and the international Canadian student organizations led to an estimation of about 3500 Canadian students enrolled in medical schools abroad.

The average annual tuition cost for a CSA ranged from C$12,250 in Poland to C$66,369 in Australia at the time of the CaRMS (2010b) survey. Site interviews revealed that international students are important revenue sources not only for the for-profit universities but also for the non-profit state universities, where CSAs' tuition supplements the national medical education costs. At the time of the CaRMS (2010b) report the median CSA debt was C$160,000 compared to the 2007 CMG median debt of C$71,000 (Merani et al., 2010). Respondents from Australia and Ireland were more successful than the respondents from the Caribbean in arranging Canadian clerkships. The vast majority (90.3%) of the respondents reported a desire to return to Canada for a portion of their postgraduate medical education, and 24.8% reported a plan to return to Canada after postgraduate training abroad. This was a significant change from the 2006 survey when only 67.2% of respondents indicated their intention to return to Canada for postgraduate training (Banner & Comeau, 2006). A similar finding in both the 2006 and 2010 survey was that the further away the respondents were from graduation, the more likely they were to respond that they intended to return to Canada (Banner & Comeau, 2006). The requirement to provide "return of service for the postgraduate training" (61.0%), their choice of discipline being difficult to obtain (57.1%), and the perception that a CSA would have difficulty matching to a program in Canada (43.8%) were cited as the main barriers regarding their return to Canada for postgraduate training. Similar to the 2006 survey, the top two career choices of CSAs in the 2010 survey were family medicine and internal medicine (Banner & Comeau, 2006). The top two university choices were the University of Toronto and the University of British Columbia.

The CaRMS (2010b) report accurately states: "This survey was based on self-reported data, which of course, lends itself to bias. At the beginning of the study, only 55 of the more than 75 schools where Canadians are now known to be studying medicine abroad were identified, as more schools are discovered every day." Interestingly, no UK schools participated in the study. Caribbean medical schools generally do not offer clerkship rotations within the Caribbean. Most clerkships are outsourced to the United States, Canada, and occasionally the United Kingdom (Canadian Resident Matching Service, 2010b). Also of note is that in countries where English is not the language spoken during communication to patients – although English may be the language used for teaching in the medical school – the communication of CSAs with the patients whom they are seeing, may be affected by the inability of the patient to communicate in English or the CSA to communicate with patients in their own language.

As a Canadian, I took the decision to study medicine abroad because the prospects of being accepted in Canada seemed quite bleak. I was very happy when I started studying medicine, consuming knowledge like I never thought possible. I however became aware of the difficulties of being accepted for residency training back in Canada halfway through medical school. Had I known how challenging it would be to obtain any residency training in Canada as an IMG, I probably wouldn't have gone abroad for my studies. I always was under pressure to outperform others, get better grades, better clerkships evaluations, and better reference letters. My record needed to be without blemishes (or very minor ones) to have any decent chance of being accepted back home. (CSA narrative, fluidsurvey)

If I could do medical school again, I would not do it any differently. I decided to go to Poland to study medicine. Because I knew of family friends that had studied in Poland, this was never a foreign idea to me although it was to my Canadian professors, friends and others. I applied to medical schools in Canada and abroad and faced much criticism regarding my Polish applications. I wanted to be a doctor and I was willing to do whatever it took to get there. Lucky for me (as it turned out), I did not get accepted to a Canadian medical school and thus I had to pursue my backup plans to go study in Poland. Not only was I getting the opportunity to study medicine but also the opportunity to live in a different culture in a beautiful city. However, studying in Poland was not all lattes and beer and travelling. School was not easy. While preparing for my Polish exams, I also had to prepare for both American and Canadian exams. While the content in all exams are the same, in Poland you are expected to know every detail of each course, and there are no "key words" to give you a hint on exams. Polish schools require you to know it all and understand it all. My curriculum mirrored what is taught in North America but we were expected to do extra classes that are part of the Polish medical curriculum. Additionally, while trying to study I wanted to take the opportunity to travel. In the four years, I was able to travel to Africa and Asia and to a majority of countries in Europe. The intensity of the medical training in Poland prepared me for the hurdles that I would have to overcome to try and make it back to Canada to do residency. As a woman in medicine, I never met any challenges because of my gender but I met challenges being labeled as an IMG (even though I am Canadian born and raised). I knew when I left for Poland it would be difficult to return to Canada for residency but it really hit me that although I would graduate as a doctor, it may take a very long time for me to actually work as a doctor in Canada, if ever. To prepare for residency applications, in my fourth year I did electives in Canada and the USA to get North American experience. In these electives I would introduce myself as a medical student and go about my duties. The residents I worked with knew I was an IMG but it usually was not until a couple of days into working with an attending doctor would they realize that I was internationally trained. This surprised me because as an IMG you assume that you are not at the same level as North American trained medical students yet in clinic these doctors could not tell the difference. This gave me hope that I might be able to get back however when you start to apply no one looks at your clinical references unless you get a desired score on a test. I scored at the requisite percentile for Canada and the USA and got interviews in both countries. American interviews were encouraging. No one cared that I was Canadian or that I studied abroad. They were impressed with my knowledge and clinical skills and actively recruited me to their program.

Canada was not the same. I had to constantly prove my knowledge of Canadian health care system and went through an intensive interview process with probing questions to evaluate my clinical skills and ability to work with others. But I did it. I matched to Canada. Relieved that my risk to study abroad paid off I did not realize that I would be labeled as an IMG for a while still. Even though I proved myself in the exams and interview process, I was still required to complete classroom training, shadowing and have a prolonged probation period to prove that I was a good fit for the Canadian health care system. I believe that obtaining clinical experience in three different countries places you to succeed best as a doctor to treat a diverse and multicultural Canadian population. I am happy to be back in Canada to do residency but I wish Canada would be more receptive to doctors returning or coming to Canada after training or working abroad. (CSA narrative, fluidsurvey)

The Literature about Female IMGs in Canada

The literature on immigrant IMGs includes very limited information on the distinction between male and female IMGs. Szafran et al. (2005) compared immigrant IMGs to Canadian (CSA) IMGs and showed that immigrant IMGs tended to be older, be married, and have dependent children. Immigrant IMGs most frequently obtained their medical education in Asia, Eastern Europe, the Middle East, or Africa, whereas Canadian IMGs (CSAs) most frequently obtained their medical degrees in Asia, the Caribbean, or Europe.

Immigrant IMGs tended to have more years of postgraduate training and clinical experience. A significantly greater proportion of immigrant IMGs perceived that there were insufficient opportunities for assessment, financial barriers to training, and licensing barriers to practise. Nearly half (45.5%) of all IMGs selected family medicine as their first choice of clinical discipline to practise in Canada. There were no significant differences between Canadian and immigrant IMGs in terms of first choice of clinical discipline (Szafran et al., 2005).

Thind and colleagues (2007) reported in 2007 that 23% of all practising physicians in Canada at that time were IMGs. Saskatchewan and Newfoundland had a higher proportion of IMG physicians (55% and 44%, respectively) than other provinces, such as Quebec. Their data suggested that IMGs tend to be older on average than CMGs and that there was a lower proportion of female physicians among IMGs.

Data from the second iteration of the CaRMS 2002 match (Crutcher et al., 2003) indicate that 72% of IMGs received their degrees from medical schools in Asia, the Middle East, or Eastern Europe, and nearly one-third had graduated since 1994 (Crutcher et al., 2003). More than half had completed their training in English, and 42% had practised medicine for one to five years before coming to Canada (Crutcher et al., 2003). The top five residency choices reported by IMGs in the 2002 CaRMS match (Crutcher et al., 2003) were family medicine and general practice (45%), internal medicine (15%), surgery (7%), obstetrics and gynecology (7%), and pediatrics (5%) (Crutcher et al., 2003). Nearly half said that their preferred practice location would be in a community of fewer than 100,000 people (Crutcher et al., 2003).

In Thind and colleagues' (2007) sample, 67% of the IMGs had received their undergraduate medical degrees from Ireland, the United Kingdom, Northern Ireland, Greece, or South Africa; 16% from developing countries (India, Iraq, China, Pakistan, the Philippines, or Egypt); 5% from eastern Europe (Poland, Bulgaria, or Romania); and the rest from the United States or Taiwan. Graduation ranged from 1955 to 2001; nearly 75% had graduated before 1983, and 95% had graduated before 1993.

The IMG physicians had more years practising in their current locations than CMGs did and were more likely to be practising solo and not to be involved in undergraduate or postgraduate teaching. While IMGs and CMGs in Thind and colleagues' (2007) study did similar numbers of deliveries and provided similar amounts of prenatal care, IMGs were less likely to provide maternity and newborn care in their practices. The IMG family physicians were more likely to be accepting new patients in their practices and were more likely to be practising in small towns or rural and isolated communities. This is an important positive contribution made by IMG physicians in providing access to primary care, especially for rural and isolated communities.

Understanding Challenges IMGs Face in Canada from the Literature

Sockalingam and colleagues (2014) conducted a survey of 35 immigrant IMGs about perceived IMG challenges during adaptation to fellowship training in Toronto. Immigrant IMGs rated their challenges from 1 (very easy) to 5 (very challenging) and these are listed below:

- Balancing professional and personal life 3. 43 ± 1. 01
- Social adjustment 2. 86 ± 1. 12

- Isolation from family 3. 37 ± 1. 29
- Communication with the interprofessional team 3. 00 ± 1. 00
- Communication with patients 2. 51 ± 1. 31
- Canadian language and slang 2. 80 ± 1. 37
- Canadian health care system 3. 09 ± 1. 07
- Local hospital system and structure 3. 49 ± 1. 01)
- Using evidence-based medicine 2. 23 ± 0. 81
- Medical documentation 3. 54 ± 1. 25
- Specialty specific clinical skills 2. 59 ± 1. 05

All the challenges agree with findings in the international immigrant IMG literature.

IMG Difficulties in Passing Canadian Certification Exams

A challenge not often mentioned by the IMG literature is the hurdle of passing the Canadian certification exams. Because it usually occurs close to the end of residency, IMGs are often very reluctant to share their failure and are often ashamed of having failed the exam. Failing the certification exam and having to repeat it can be extremely stressful for IMGs. There is an increasing number of IMGs taking the College of Family Physicians of Canada (CFPC) certification examination, and IMGs now represent about 30% of the candidates (Walsh et al., 2011). There are two routes to the CFPC certification examination for IMGs, one through practice eligibility and the other through a residency program.

There is a complex and detailed selection process for IMGs into family medicine residency programs and detailed requirements for the practice eligibility route. Despite this, the success rate for all IMGs in Canadian family medicine residency programs on the CFPC certification exam is significantly lower than for CMGs, and has been decreasing over time. In 2007 CMGs' overall success rate on the CFPC exam was 90.4%, whereas the success rate for IMGs was 66.0%. In 2008, the pass rate was 74% for residency-trained IMGs. In 2009, it was 64%, and, in 2010, there was a 51% success rate. A similar pattern was reflected in IMGs coming from a practice eligible route (non-residency trained) but with much higher failure rates (Walsh et al., 2011).

On the examinations of the Royal College of Physicians and Surgeons of Canada (RCPSC), the relative success rates between IMGs and graduates of Canadian medical schools is less striking, but still different. From 2005 to 2009, for candidates on their first attempt, the CMG pass rate for primary specialty examinations was 95%, while the IMG pass rate was 76%; for subspecialty examinations, the success rates were 96% and 75%, respectively. There are a number of differences between the two specialty colleges. The training time for the RCPSC is at least double that of the CFPC programs, and the RCPSC includes graduates of US Liaison Committee on Medical Education accredited medical schools in their IMG numbers, although there are only a small number of US graduates (Walsh et al., 2011).

Common Themes Identified by IMGs Accompanied by Narratives

In this section of the chapter, narratives written by IMGs are used to demonstrate barriers and facilitators identified by IMGs. Narratives were obtained by sending out an email from the author to IMGs she had worked with over the years with a link to an anonymous fluid survey to respond to with a narrative. The email explained that their anonymous responses would be used to "speak for IMGs" in a chapter on female IMGs in a book about women in medicine. The IMGs were also encouraged to forward the email to another female IMG they might think would want to contribute. Eligible participants were IMGs who were currently enrolled in a training program in Ontario or had completed their Canadian residency within 10 years of the start of the study. Narratives from the AFMC IMG modules were also quoted, as well as narratives from the IMG literature.

Common themes were identified by immigrant IMGs from their narratives.

Difficulties Gaining Acceptance into a Medical Training Program (Training Entry Barriers)

Wong and Lohfeld (2008) report that this issue was typical of many IMGs experiences, primarily stemming from a disproportionately small number of IMG training positions despite the continuing doctor shortages in Canada. Many IMGs described the admissions process as logistically difficult, impersonal, and stressful as a result of ambiguous selection criteria and lack of feedback (Wong & Lohfeld, 2008).

My postgraduate training (twice as long as the average Canadian GP) was irrelevant, I was told that I would have to repeat my residency. All these requests made me feel like I was some dishonest quack, trying to sneak into the superlative Canadian system. That system repeatedly proclaimed its desire and intent to uphold the high quality health care it provided to its citizens. I was merely a landed immigrant, definitely a second class citizen. From where I stood, I felt like I was on Ellis Island, being inspected for deadly diseases, begging for entry, suspected of becoming a parasite on this perfect society. (AFMC, 2006)

I believe the journey of immigration begins far before landing time and an important factor that affects achievement as an IMG is the experience one carries in her backpack on arrival. Fortunately, besides being a clinician I had research and management experiences from back home that helped me find a research assistance job soon after arriving. I think this early start helped me enormously with better understanding of the health system, enhancing my communication skills, connecting to people and integrating to the new environment. Also, I applied for a Master's degree as soon as I found a supportive supervisor and could define a project in an area I had passion for. My goal was enrolment in a residency program, so I needed to study for the MCC exams but I was pursuing my graduate studies to PhD and post-doc level at the same time to make an academic job available; as plan B. I should confess that sometimes I felt anxious when comparing myself with many other IMG friends who were spending most of their time in the libraries studying hard for the exams. Keeping myself busy with other activities helped me a lot to cope with all the stress at that time and kept my mood tuned! I was hopeful and determined to pursue my clinical career but knew in case of failure, the future wouldn't be that dark and other career options would be up there for me. I believe having a plan B and engaging in supplementary activities gave me a peace of mind and helped me a lot in ending up with my plan A, which was entering a residency program through IMG stream. (Canadian female IMG narrative, fluidsurvey)

I came without my husband when I immigrated to Canada in 2001, with four children, and my youngest was less than 4 years old. However, I was still lucky enough to have the financial support of my husband throughout my journey. I was lucky in this way because I knew many other IMGs who had to work to support themselves and their families financially while preparing for exams. I was struggling not only because I was an IMG, but also because I was a mother with 4 children in a completely new and foreign country. With much determination, persistence, and hope I was able to do all what one can possibly do. The journey was difficult and long; obstacles were here and there. I experienced failure at some times, and success at other times. Anyways, I fulfilled all the requirements by 2005, and then I started to apply to different programs through CARMS. Finally, by 2008, I received an invitation for an interview, and that was the day I had been waiting for throughout my journey. Luckily, I was accepted from the one and only invitation I received. It was the family medicine program. I was happy with the news as University is very close to where I was living at the time, in addition to it being an excellent program. I found that everything was moving very fast as soon as I started the program. I found genuine and great support. Everyone in the program was trying to help me. My final message to IMGs: do not give up, as long as you keep trying, you are going to get there. There is always light at the end of the tunnel. (IMG narrative, fluidsurvey)

What I think that could be better is when you try to transition to a clinical fellowship, especially because of all the [licensing body] and licensing procedures and translations and so many people you have to talk with to get the license done … So, one thing is that the license is really hard to get, in my opinion. It's a very bureaucratic process, and all. (Sockalingam et al., 2014)

Loss

Loss was a common theme early in IMGs' training. Wong and Lohfeld (2008) described the IMG experience as having three phases: loss, disorientation professionally and personally, and adaptation. IMGs experienced loss in the personal domain (loss of personal identity, belonging, financial autonomy, and ability to fulfil familial roles) and the professional domain (loss of professional identity and status, as well as professional devaluation (Wong & Lohfeld, 2008).

You felt dehumanised, in a sense, as if you had lost something that you had already achieved) that [your profession] had been taken away from you. You had to sort of work to get it back. (Wong & Lohfeld, 2008, p. 56)

Loss in the personal domain was often expressed in the form of personal sacrifices that took their toll on family members and marital relations (Wong & Lohfeld, 2008).

The reason for being in Canada is intimately tied up with the experience of being an IMG. As physicians, we have all learnt to postpone gratification. The majority of those I met were here to provide a better future for their families, to raise them in a just and peaceful society, where human rights are respected. Some were opportunists, hoping to make a better living than back home. They were all prepared to put up with a certain amount of hardship in order to achieve these goals. The visible hardships included poverty, alienation from loved ones, under-employment, and loss of religious and cultural opportunities. The hidden hardship was putting up with these difficult feelings of frustration, anger, mixed with uncertainty and hopefulness. We had all heard of somebody who had succeeded in establishing themselves as respected physicians, and of others who made pragmatic decisions to retrain in more available specialties. Many entered the program as surgeons, not knowing if they had a chance to become licensed as surgeons, or whether they would have to choose pathology or family medicine if there were no other opportunities. They entered not knowing if they would be living with family in Toronto, or whether they would be expected to leave for Ottawa at short notice. Some marriages suffered, some failed. For many, the price of the choices made, was high. (AFMC, 2006)

Disorientation

Disorientation in IMGs' professional and personal lives was also a frequent occurrence in the early months of their training. Participants described "feeling like aliens" (Wong & Lohfeld, 2008, p. 56).

> Uncertainty over how to properly conduct themselves around peers and staff supervisors. Professional role confusion resulted from problems with understanding the expected roles and responsibilities of IMGs within the medical hierarchy, and cross-national differences in medical practice. Confusion also arose over the contextual areas of practice, such as the organizational features of the Canadian medical system, the use of medical technology and therapies, the scope of practice, doctor–patient and inter-professional relationships, and medico--legal and ethical issues. (Wong & Lohfeld, 2008, p. 56)

The transition from practicing Third World medicine to practicing First World medicine is one of the biggest jumps that I have made in terms of my practice career. (Wong & Lohfeld, 2008)

I come from a culture where it's a virtue to be modest and humble... whereas here, that can easily be misinterpreted as ignorance or worse, stupidity. (Wong & Lohfeld, 2008, p. 56)

Socio-cultural differences also added to IMGs' sense of disorientation. Some female IMGs who have never had a driver's licence or never had to drive suddenly find themselves in a residency program where a driver's licence is essential to meet the requirements of residency training. For some IMGs it is their first experience of working on an electronic medical record or practising evidence-based medicine. The majority of participants in Sockalingam and colleagues' (2014) study described their initial experience in fellowship as "a shock phase" or period of disorientation that accompanies moving into a new country and culture. Most fellows felt disoriented and disconnected during the process of integration into novel personal and professional roles within a new healthcare system in a North American educational and training environment (Sockalingam et al., 2014).

Adaptation

We have to first settle down, get used to Canada, get to know the process and examinations, settle down our families and kids first before being able to focus on requirements of the selection process. Finances is also a challenge and finding any job for as means of support is important and all of this leads to time passing by and effecting our chances of being selected. (IMG narrative, fluidsurvey)

I think settling into a new country is probably the biggest challenge.... As I say, I'm married with a young boy, so moving everybody over, and I'm trying to get my [young] boy into a sleep pattern again – that was pretty challenging. But, I'm getting settled into a new apartment. Finding your way around the city, I think they were probably the biggest challenges. (Sockalingam et al., 2014)

I would like program directors to be aware that for a female IMG it's not only the work that is in a new environment but also it a big change in life – where you live, families moving, young kids to be taken care of without much support here. (IMG narrative, fluidsurvey)

Wong and Lohfeld's (2008) participants described several coping strategies IMGs used to adapt to their new situation. These strategies included trying to blend in with their Canadian peers, staying out of trouble, and various psychological defence mechanisms such as "telling myself that this was a necessary evil ... in order to keep an optimistic attitude," reframing the training as a temporary detour or an opportunity to learn new skills, and trying to stay focused on long-term goals. Participants identified three factors that helped their adjustment. The first of these was support from designated faculty mentors for IMGs; the second was peer support from other IMGs in training; and the third was sufficient time spent in the training program (Wong & Lohfeld, 2008).

Balancing Personal and Professional Life

I immigrated to Canada 8 years ago with my husband and two young kids. I completed a PhD and a residency training during this time. I have been extremely fortunate as I met with great people along the way who supported and mentored me. The biggest challenge for me was balancing my professional and personal life. It was incredibly hard to find time for my family during my residency training due to increasing demands on residents time and lack of support/accommodation for women with children.

The biggest challenge I had and still have as a female IMG physician has been to keep a balance between my family life and professional life. Many of us female IMGs start our career building in Canada in a stage of life that we have children and established families. This limits the time necessary to focus on our career compared to our Canadian counterparts who are typically younger and in earlier stages of life with less responsibilities. (Canadian IMG narrative, fluidsurvey)

Cultural Adjustment

Hall et al. (2004) states that, for example, a woman IMG is expected to be quiet and shy in her own culture. This could be misinterpreted by her Canadian colleagues as being unhappy or as lacking confidence. With this perspective in mind, issues related to gender, power/hierarchy structures, differences in work ethics, expectations of degrees of autonomy in practice, responsibilities, and accountability could be more directly addressed with IMGs during orientation.

> IMGs have practiced in settings where disease patterns, treatment options, health care delivery and workplace hierarchies differ from their new environment. These differences can cause stress as IMGs try to understand the reality of practice in their adopted country, where parenting traditions,

sexual roles and acceptable behaviour may differ from those in their home countries (Huijskens et al., 2010, p. 796).

Cultural adjustment is another challenge that many of us encounter. Therefore, the level of eventual success or achievements strongly depends on the level of resilience and management skills in a high demanding, multi-task situation. Like many other female IMG fellows, life has been really exhausting for me at many points! However, I always remind myself that I have immigrated for a better and higher quality life; life is going on and it will never wait for me to finish my challenges to enjoy it! Therefore, I try to mindfully enjoy every day of my life by reminding myself of what I have achieved so far, finding joy in my work and spending quality time with my family despite my limited time. (IMG narrative, fluidsurvey)

Starting over at a Later Age Than Canadian Graduates

You start a residency picked from the limited basket for the "beggars who cannot be choosers"...So you concentrate on making the absolute best out of your residency. You realize what a privilege it is to be able to work as a resident again where you have access to situations with your current knowledge and previous experience so that you can learn at your particular level... You have lost 10 years of income and career growth opportunity. (AFMC, 2006)

Many of us female IMGs start our career building in Canada in a stage of life that we have children and established families. This limits the time necessary to focus on our career compared to our Canadian counterparts who are typically younger and in earlier stages of life with less responsibilities. (IMG narrative, fluidsurvey)

The Need to Be Resilient

Therefore, the level of eventual success or achievements strongly depends on the level of resilience and management skills in a high demanding, multi-task situation. Like many other female IMG fellows, life has been really exhausting for me at many points!

However, I always remind myself that I have immigrated for a better and higher quality life; life is going on and it will never wait for me to finish my challenges to enjoy it!

Therefore, I try to mindfully enjoy every day of my life by reminding myself of what I have achieved so far, finding joy in my work and spending quality time with my family despite my limited time. (IMG narrative, fluidsurvey)

The Need for Planning

I attribute a large proportion of my success to good planning. I was in medical school when my family moved to Canada I realized that I should do my post grad training there. I had the benefit of this forewarning. I carefully planned my electives around Canada and arranged my Canadian board exams so that I would be ready to apply for the 2014 match as soon as I graduate in the fall of 2013. I think that female IMGs have some unique challenges. Many are not free to relocate anywhere they match as their families already have roots in certain cities. Some have young children to care for along the difficult process of applying for the match. I was rather unique that I had no such struggles. I was young and unattached so I could literally go where the wind would take me. It was very important to me to get my training from an excellent university and a strong program.

Geography was not an issue. The biggest challenge that I faced was discouragement from all sides that I was on a suicide mission. That matching in Canada is impossible and that I was being a fool wasting time and money applying here. That I should just apply to the US like every one else. No one understood my reasons for applying to Canada and that environment of criticism and self doubt really made it a hard time for me. My family helped me through it by reminding me that just because statistically chances were slim did not mean it was impossible. I believed in my competence and made it. (IMG narrative, fluidsurvey)

Financial Challenges

Finances is also a challenge and finding any job for a means of support is important and all of this leads to time passing by and effecting our chances of being selected. It would help if the greater challenges that IMG immigrants go through are realized and measures are taken to specifically help them. (IMG narrative, fluidsurvey)

I was still lucky enough to have the financial support of my husband throughout my journey. I was lucky in this way because I knew many other IMGs who had to work to support themselves and their families financially while preparing for exams. (IMG narrative, fluidsurvey)

IMGs have to sit several expensive exams as part of their journey to admission into postgraduate residency programs or obtaining a licence to practise in a new country. As IMGs, CSAs pay much higher tuition fees than the local medical students, and CSAs often complete medical school with more than C$200,000 of study debt. As noted earlier, the CSA median debt is C$160,000 compared to the 2007 CMG median debt of C$71,000 (Canadian Resident Matching Service, 2010b).

Immigrant IMGs have to support themselves and their families while completing all the costly exams and courses before trying to access the Canadian system. Because IMGs start earning much later in their careers, they often are not financially secure to retire.

You have lost ten years of income and career growth opportunity. (AFMC, 2006)

Discrimination and Harassment

I am an IMG and I must say the transition was difficult. Not because of the challenges in performing your tasks but because of the constant 'under the microscope' approach of the program director who themselves are uncomfortable seeing IMG with more than adequate experience become senior medical residents within a few months. It is some kind of a bias they may have which they need to get over with. It would only help if they were more supportive. Although, I must add in my experience I have met the most encouraging colleagues and staff in the same first few months that helped me get past the initial stressful stumbling block. I would like program directors to be aware that for a female IMG it's not only the work that is in a new environment but also it is a big change in life – where you live, families moving, young kids to be taken care of without much support here. I am sure the program directors have their own viewpoint and experiences that they look back on but they need to be less judgmental and more helpful to help through the first few months. (IMG narrative, fluidsurvey)

Respondents to a survey estimated that approximately one third of IMG fellows experienced discrimination related to being an IMG (fellows, 30%; supervisors, 37%). Nearly 49% of fellows and 54% of supervisors favoured fellowship supervisors undergoing diversity training (Sockalingam et al., 2014).

The most surprising thing about Canadian culture is the receptiveness that Canadians have to foreigners. They are welcoming to foreigners. (Sockalingam et al., 2014)

I think it's basically Torontonians and this place is built on a multilayered culture, so very few people I think discriminate against. I feel very comfortable in Toronto and in the hospital. (Sockalingam et al., 2014)

Need for Feedback

Several IMG fellows reported challenges feeling disconnected with the educational system and a sense of isolation as a trainee:

Nobody has asked me if I'm happy with what I'm doing ... nobody told me if they're happy with what I'm doing, so ... I think, it's not structured in a way to give feedback and receive feedback. (Sockalingam et al., 2014)

Mentors

I would like to thank some of the mentors who themselves were IMG's who guided me through this process. I have met the most amazing people since being here and I am glad I made the decision to come here and not listen to all the negative discouraging stories that we hear most of the time when we contemplate beginning this process. (IMG narrative, fluidsurvey)

Participants indicated that they received the most academic and moral support from senior international students and their international peers and mentors (Malau-Aduli, 2011).

Honestly, I think having people who have been there and done that helps a lot, they're able to advise us on things to do and things not to do. (Malau-Aduli, 2011)

Not Causing Shame to Family Members back Home

IMG participants in a study by Malau-Aduli (2011) indicated that they had at some stage in their pursuit of the medical degree, considered withdrawing, and this was due to the challenges of the medical education (stress and workload). However, "withdrawal isn't considered as an option because of the shame and unhappiness it would cause my family members" (Malau-Aduli, 2011, p. 6).

Participants concentrated on the positive outcomes of the process and the prestige attached to completing the medical degree (Malau-Aduli, 2011).

Working in a Multicultural Canada Requires IMGs

A lot has been said about the importance of integrating IMGs in the health care system of Canada. I will give you another reason.

While doing my ER rotation during my residency I saw a 6-year-old girl with an upper respiratory tract infection symptoms with suspected otitis media. She was accompanied by her harried dad with her five other siblings. All were younger than her (the youngest about six months old), in various stages of URTI themselves. The family had recently emigrated from Afghanistan and had language issues. When I went back to see her, she, along with her Dad, had gone to see her Mom … in the Emergency Psychiatry Unit!

In the Emergency Psychiatry Unit, I witnessed a tense situation. Dad was shouting loudly in his broken English, above his wailing kids: "You can't take wife away; I can't take care of kids." The psychiatry resident was dialing the Children's Aid Society (CAS) number. Assessing the situation, I asked the resident to hold the call for 10 minutes while I talked to the person. Having knowledge of his language and culture, I asked him if he understood what was happening. He only knew that his wife had no "illness," sure she was a bit down after her last baby and threatened to commit suicide, but he could take care of her at home, he could stop her from killing herself. Besides she had the house keys, how will he get back in?

In his language, I explained postpartum depression, how it was a real illness, how he could not prevent her suicide and how she needed emergency treatment. I also explained the role of CAS, how by law they can remove the kids if they think he cannot take care of them. I was able to get his house keys back, have some family members stay with him for a while and arrange for him to see his wife the next day. Thus, the matter was amicably resolved. I was able to save a family the trauma of separation and the tax payers' money by avoiding the need for CAS involvement. And this was only because I was at the right place at the right time.

This incident made me aware that for the ever-expanding multicultural population of Canada we need a multicultural health force, hence the need for IMGs. (AFMC, 2006)

Communication Skills

I think one of the weakest point[s] in our country is [that] they don't teach you much about how to interact with a patient, as they do here. We just learned by [spending] two years in the clinic. (Dorgan et al., 2009)

What emerged from Dorgan and colleagues' (2009) study was that the overall lack of communication training seemed to have emotional and behavioural consequences for many IMGs. For example, some reported that they had experienced confusion related to communication training and assessment on entering their residency programs, because they had never experienced such pedagogical techniques.

We have three years of basic science, which is anatomy [and] physiology, and, after that, we have one year…where we learn particularly about the disease and diagnosis. (Dorgan et al., 2009)

Dorgan et al. (2009) states: "One barrier to cross-cultural communication with patients was that IMGs had not studied communications in their foreign medical training, a finding similar to previous research."

You have to learn on your own. You have to observe how this doctor is approaching the patient. We were not taught by specific lectures. (Dorgan et al., 2009)

According to this same participant, this lack of formal training seemed to extend to "zero education" about how to communicate with patients and families about such issues as death and dying (Dorgan et al., 2009).

Isolation

IMGs often feel isolated, and women IMGs have unique stresses.

Leaving Canada to pursue my medical education was not an easy decision to make. I left behind everyone I knew and moved to a town where I knew no one. I was scared at first but over time, my confidence grew and I established a deeper connection with myself.

Medical school was a wonderful time where I travelled around the United States of America doing my clinical rotations. It seemed like I was just getting used to one city when I had to move to another. It was difficult to meet people outside of the hospital and foster close relationships. At the time, it didn't seem to matter because we were all in the same boat. Sleep-hospital-eat-sleep. Repeat. I was fortunate enough to land a residency in Canada. I am now back in my hometown, close to my friends and family. Although I am home, I often feel lonelier than I did in medical school. There is more work, less time to study, and not enough time to spend with family and friends. (CSA narrative, fluidsurvey)

Family is very important as well but since they are so far away, there really isn't much they can do apart from encouraging us I guess. (Malau-Aduli, 2011)

I call home once a week as I can make cheap overseas calls to my family and friends. (Malau-Aduli, 2011)

Some IMGs reported being homesick and missing their country and relatives (Huijskens et al., 2010). Loneliness and isolation are issues for many IMGs in practice. In some provinces IMGs have to sign a five-year underserviced area agreement, which often leads to the IMG being separated from her family and cultural community.

Thind and colleagues' (2007) study demonstrated that compared with CMGs, IMGs had been in practice longer at their current locations and were more likely to be in solo practice and accepting new patients, but were less likely to be providing maternity and newborn care. They were also more likely to be serving small towns and rural and isolated communities.

It is ironic that although IMGs are recognized as an important resource to reduce doctor shortages, they still face significant training entry barriers and challenges in becoming fully integrated in their new professional communities. This discrepancy may be reduced if IMGs were to be more highly valued and better integrated as full members of the medical community, rather than perceived simply as an available labour source. (Wong & Lohfeld, 2008)

Terry and colleagues (2014) reported the same professional isolation among IMGs practising in Rural Tasmania.

Gender

One IMG stated:

Some of them [male residents] do not want women to work. Some of them think women should stay at home. We have an internal struggle that we should say we are here, we exist and a male making you feel that you should go home. (Hall et al., 2004)

Cultural

I think it's a very different experience because when you are in psychotherapy… you know, I think you feel more confident about what you have to do because if you are doing Psychodynamic Therapy you need to take into account the culture, right? Like what is appropriate for this culture and how families … you know, what are families like in Canada? So, let's say, you know, you have shared custody … you have a lot of things that plays into families here that I don't have back in [country of origin] – not that common. So, I had to adapt, I would say … for me it was like, as you know, a big cultural experience when I have to shift to a different culture. (Sockalingam et al., 2014)

People in my culture, they don't want to know a lot about their problems, especially if they are dying … Tell the family. (Hall et al., 2004)

We don't have enough information about how your system is run … We don't have social workers … We don't have to spend time doing [paperwork] … We just discharge people and that's it. (Hall et al., 2004)

An international graduate has difficulty in merging with the new atmosphere in all branches, but this is particularly extreme in medicine, where the nature of practice is very sensitive and personal. The difficulties I personally encountered are mostly cultural, especially coming from an Eastern conservative environment, and to a much less extent different medical context, in following Canadian guidelines in approaching different diseases.

An example of a cultural issue I faced during my family medicine rotation was to meet and examine a transgendered patient, previously a male, now a female. When my supervisor introduced the issue to me, I couldn't imagine myself seeing the patient or even talking to her. I felt this was an awkward and uncomfortable situation, which I had never experienced before. I even asked my supervisor frankly not to see this patient. She was very understanding and calmed me down a lot. She suggested that I take my time to calm down and see the patient first from the camera before going in the exam room. She then went in with me to introduce me to the patient to help in melting the ice. She then left the room and I gradually started to ease up and at the end found the visit successful. My supervisor was ready with her feedback after viewing the interview through the camera.

This was an example of a cultural problem that was solved by the help of an understanding supervisor. I think international medical graduates need lots of support from all staff: physicians, nurses, social workers and all members of the medical team. This is to minimize problems and conflicts arising at the introduction to the Canadian system, without which the help could take a much longer time. (AFMC, 2006)

Family/Children Responsibilities

This theme related to balancing personal and professional life.

Many of us female IMGs start our career building in Canada in a stage of life that we have children and established families. This limits the time necessary to focus on our career compared to our Canadian counterparts who are typically younger and in earlier stages of life with less responsibilities. Therefore, I try to mindfully enjoy every day of my life by reminding myself of what I have achieved so far, finding joy in my work and spending quality time with my family despite my limited time. (IMG narrative, fluidsurvey)

Being Labelled as an IMG

As a woman in medicine I never met any challenges because of my gender but I met challenges being labelled as an IMG (even though I am Canadian born and raised).

I knew when I left for Poland it would be difficult to return to Canada for residency but it really hit me that although I would graduate as a doctor, it may take a very long time for me to actually work as a doctor in Canada, if ever. To prepare for residency applications, in my fourth year I did electives in Canada and the USA to get North American experience. In these electives I would introduce myself as a medical student and go about my duties. The residents I worked with knew I was an IMG but it usually was not until a couple of days into working with an attending doctor would they realize that I was internationally trained. This surprised me because as an IMG you assume that you are not at the same level as North American trained medical students yet in clinic these doctors could not tell the difference. This gave me hope that I might be able to get back however when you start to apply no one looks at your clinical references unless you get a desired score on a test. I scored at the requisite percentile for Canada and the USA and got interviews in both countries. American interviews were encouraging. No one cared that I was Canadian or that I studied abroad. They were impressed with my knowledge and clinical skills and actively recruited me to their program. Canada was not the same. I had to constantly prove my knowledge of Canadian health care system and went through an intensive interview process with probing questions to evaluate my clinical skills and ability to work with others. But I did it. I matched to Canada.

Relieved that my risk to study abroad paid off I did not realize that I would be labelled as an IMG for a while still. Even though I proved myself in the exams and interview process, I was still required to complete classroom training, shadowing and have a prolonged probation period to prove that I was a good fit for the Canadian health care system. I believe that obtaining clinical experience in three different countries places you to succeed best as a doctor to treat a diverse and multicultural Canadian population. I am happy to be back in Canada to do residency but I wish Canada would be more receptive to doctors returning or coming to Canada after training or working abroad. (CSA narrative, fluidsurvey)

Relationships

I certainly feel the cultural pressures on a daily basis to now settle down and start my own family. To be honest, I really would love for that to happen. Unfortunately, there is little time to meet men. The men I do meet seem to be very interested in the fact that I am a doctor. I occasionally will meet a man who confesses he would never be able to be in a relationship with a woman who earns more money than him and I never see him again. The men who see past the salary are deterred after I mention that I am obligated to serve the province in an under-serviced area for five years after I graduate. They don't want someone they will see once or twice a month. They want a commitment. And I agree with them because that is what I want as well. So here I am, waiting for that moment where I can put myself before my career. Only time will tell what the future holds for me. (CSA narrative, fluidsurvey)

Previous Traumatic Experiences

Previous traumatic experiences were specifically identified as barriers by some IMGs, and some IMGs reported reliving traumatic experiences during work in psychiatry (Huijskens et al., 2010). IMGs who arrived as refugees from war-torn countries to Canada, often also had to deal with consequences of trauma in their families, such as a female IMG whose daughter suffered from mutism after witnessing war atrocities.

Language

Oral presentations, reflective pieces, essays, and written assignments are often experienced as stressful by IMGs

As we often got stuck with word choices and need to translate the meaning of words in our heads before expressing them, an arduous time consuming task. (Sockalingam et al., 2014)

IMG residents who do not speak English as their first language may struggle with idioms, nuances, and vernacular terms. Limited understanding of such terms in medical team-based settings may lead to communication breakdowns, which are a major cause of adverse events (Sockalingam et al., 2014).

I was born, raised and educated in two different countries outside Canada where neither English nor French were the official languages.

Once I had finished my medical school, I immigrated to Canada to reunite with my family who was already established in Canada. My English at that point was very rudimentary. Subsequently, I had spent the first year in Canada improving my English by taking several ESL (English as Second Language) classes. The preparatory work for the IMG paid off three years after when I was selected among the 24 candidates to start the clerkship.

As I am writing and reflecting upon my overall IMG experience, I have realized that it was mostly positive and enjoyable. I felt well accepted among my fellow students and later residents as well as staff physicians, nurses and faculties. The impression I had was that I was always treated as an equal to a Canadian graduate. Naturally, I am an optimist but I have chosen to share the only improper incident that took place at the end of my residency training.

It was late at night on the L & D (Labour and Delivery) ward after a long regular clinical day. My nulliparous patient had entered the active phase of labour. At that level of training I had to closely follow and check her as the labour progressed and report to my attending who was on his way to the hospital. Since it was the same ward where I did my Obstetrics during the clerkship a few years back, one of the nurses recognized me and started a very jovial conversation about my future plans, being that I was at the end of the residency. She was curious to know if I would pursue Obstetrics as a Family Practitioner and where were my intentions to practise medicine. I had replied that I would try a rather adventurous route to perhaps even practise for a while in Australia. Another nurse had overheard our dialogue and sarcastically commented that Aussies, themselves, speak English and began to laugh…Her implying that my English was insufficient made me go over almost every word I said that night and day. Although I was tired and maybe my pronunciation was a bit deficient, I didn't feel that the other nurse had difficulties understanding me. In all that shock I had managed to reply that I do speak, write and read in three languages and that since English in not my mother tongue, it may sound a bit rusty. We had stopped there.

However, the inspiring experiences in my IMG training have far outweighed this one. (AFMC, 2006)

Implications of Having to Sign an Underserviced Area Agreement

In several provinces, IMGs have to sign a five-year underserviced agreement after residency training in Canada or are only eligible for a licence restricted to an underserviced area when entering Canada.

On Struggling to Pass College Certification Exams

As referred to before in this chapter, the pass rates for IMGs on college certification exams in Canada are significantly lower than for Canadian medical graduates. This is a huge cause of stress, embarrassment, and shame for many IMGs. In the worse scenario this can end in the IMG leaving the country after not being able to pass the exam in the allowed number of attempts (MacLellan et al., 2010; Walsh et al., 2011). Analyses revealed that country of study and performance on the MCC evaluating examination are among the predictors of performance on the CFPC and the RCPSC certification examinations. Of interest, the analyses also suggest discipline-specific relationships between previous professional experience and examination success (Schabort et al., 2014).

IMGs More Prone to Attract Complaints to Medical Boards and Adverse Disciplinary Findings

Elkin and colleagues' (2012) Australian data showed that IMGs are more likely than Australian-trained doctors to attract complaints to medical boards and adverse disciplinary findings, but the risks differ markedly by country of training. Complaints were higher against IMGs than non-IMGs (odds ratio [OR], 1.24; 95% CI, 1.13–1.36; $p < .001$), as were the odds of adverse disciplinary findings (OR, 1.41; 95% CI, 1.07–1.85; $p = .01$). However, disaggregation of IMGs into their countries of qualification showed wide variation between countries with ORs as high as 4.02 (OR, 4.02; 95% CI, 2.38–6.77) for certain countries of training, but IMGs from some of the other countries examined had odds that were not significantly different from Australian-trained doctors.

The study by Papadakis et al. (2008) did not show this trend in IMGs who completed postgraduate training in Canada or the United States. Tamblyn and colleagues (2007), however, did find that scores achieved in patient-physician communication and clinical decision making on a national licensing examination predicted complaints to medical regulatory authorities in the United States and Canada and practice in primary care (Tamblyn et al., 2002).

I got an opportunity to be trained in a bit more relaxed environment where you can practise a lot … it means, that learning certain techniques and performing more complicated trials, it was a bit easier … I said my advantage was doing that and practising that in an environment that was not threatened with litigation and of course I changed my practice here when I realized that … that was the way how to go [here].

You are completely covered by litigation guidelines, by the protocols and the things, and you change your practice, starting to do the same things as, ahh … but … I still think that that is defensive medicine, not exactly the right way to go, but that's the way. (Harris, 2014, pp. 259–82)

Mental Health Issues

Sockalingam and colleagues' (2014) reported that dominant society immersion, junior residency training level, and poor social supports have been associated with lower mental health in IMG residents, underscoring the need for greater support with the transition process.

Working in an Interdisciplinary Team

I think that here in Canada the differences between doctors and nurses and whoever else are less than in [country of previous medical training] ... it's much more prominent, the difference between like, the group of doctors and the group of receptionists and the group of nurses and ... and here it's better, actually like everybody's like ... part of the same team and you feel that it's just that you're part of a team and everybody's the same and like, there's no difference between any of us. (Sockalingam et al., 2014)

CEAs (CSAs) Competing with Immigrant IMGs for IMG Stream Positions

One overall experience I would like to share is highlighting the difference between the experiences for IMGs and Canadians Educated Abroad (CEA). I would like to note that the changes being brought into the system, and other new supports being introduced are aimed at CEA than IMGs. Majority of residents being selected are CEAs and not immigrant IMGs. If there is a clear distinction made between the two then that would highlight the different experiences and more challenges that IMGs have overcome than CEAs: moving to Canada, starting over in a new surroundings, having to sit several exams. more (often even passing all LMCC examinations before obtaining a residency), being questioned about our command of the English Language all the time. This despite the fact that many immigrant IMGs have had extensive training and hands-on practice which can be an asset to the healthcare system. It is also hard for IMGs to often meet the rule/preference of being out of practice under 2 years because we have to first settle down, get used to Canada, get to know the process and examinations, settle down our families and kids first before being able to focus on requirements of the selection process. Finances is also a challenge and finding any job for as means of support is important and all of this leads to time passing by and affecting our chances of being selected. It would help if the greater challenges that IMG immigrants go through are realized and measures are taken to specifically help them. Thanks. (IMG narrative, fluidsurvey)

Suggestions on How to Address the Challenges Faced by IMGs

From an IMG

DEAR IMG PRECEPTORS

I have thought of a few things that might help in the teaching and learning of IMG residents in our program. Foremost is the fact that we need to be understood, and tolerated in certain situations due to not knowing the system, rather than a lack of clinical knowledge. We come with a past and a lot of family responsibilities.

The first thing that comes to my mind is that preceptors should take time to review the IMG residents' personal information, background and experience before they start residency. For example, some of them might have worked 10–15 years as a gynaecologist, radiologist, or paediatrician. Their clinical experience is different from an IMG who graduated in the Dominican Republic, and came here directly to enter as an IMG.

The use of the English language is also different in other parts of the world, even in medical terminology, such as how to describe an illness.

Our knowledge base is very wide to get into the program we are studying to complete, so standards are extremely high. And the entry OSCEs are tougher than any I have done in this program. This meant that when we enter the program, our base knowledge is different, which affects our clinical practice. Evidence-based medicine and research is something that we need to be encouraged to learn about, so we know how to treat and diagnose, but presenting a case will be different from a Canadian graduate. That at times is frustrating for both teacher and the resident – it also affects our evaluations.

Another interesting point is that we come from a system where there is a respect for our seniors, which runs hand in hand with the formality of addressing tutors or seniors with their title and last name. Not only does it take us time to get used being on a first name basis, it sometimes makes the working environment hard or uncomfortable. If the preceptors meet the IMG candidate before, or in the initial few weeks of residency and find out what their concerns are, and explain certain things, the work environment can improve considerably.

It is important to note that 80% of IMG graduates come into the program already having completed the LMCC II exam – so their approach to learning is very different … my thought is that they need less didactic teaching and more clinical work. More is needed about how to refer patients to services (e.g. physio, social work, specialists, worker's compensation etc.) and what expectations are regarding other health care professionals such as nurses, lab techs, social workers, etc.

There are several other issues. IMGs know how to prescribe and what to prescribe but might not understand how the prescription is written here. Computer systems and data entry can be a challenge.

Finally, behavioural science tutorials are a great challenge. Most IMGs have never videotaped themselves before, or been in discussions focused on interview skills.

Therefore, our contributions in such programs are different from regular graduates. Maybe these teachers could try to approach teaching in multidimensional methods so the IMGs can have an increasing role in behavioural science tutorials. (AFMC, 2006)

From the Literature

Hall and colleagues (2004) conducted a needs assessment to assess Canadian IMGs communication skills needs through focus groups, surveys, and interviews with IMGs, program directors, allied health professionals, and experts in communication skills. They concluded that IMGs required a combination of language skills, teaching on how to get things done in the health care system, opportunities to practise specific skills, support systems, and faculty and staff education on the cultural challenges faced by IMGs.

Wong & Lohfeld (2008) identified three factors that helped IMG adjustment. The first of these was support from designated faculty mentors for IMGs; the second was peer support from other IMGs in training; and the third was sufficient time spent in the training program.

A qualitative study by Curran et al. (2008) conducted telephone interviews of IMGs and senior administrators of medical services in Newfoundland and Labrador. The importance of reflecting on one's own cultural bias and learning and integrating into a new community were key findings. Orientation and mentoring were felt to be important to this, as well as in reducing professional isolation.

A systematic review by Pilotto and colleagues (2007) identified key issues for clinicians training IMGs for their medical workforce. Five areas were identified as high level for the clinician teacher: the need for IMGs to adjust to a change in status; for clinicians to understand the high level of language skills required by IMGs; the importance of developing IMGs' skills in communicating with patients; the need to understand IMGs' expectations about teaching and learning; and finally the need for IMGs to be able to interact effectively with a range of people.

A study by MacLellan et al. (2010) examined the success of IMGs in postgraduate family medicine training on the pre-residency Collège des médecins du Québec medical clinical sciences written examination and objective structured clinical examination, as well as the post-residency CFPC certification examination. Although IMGs were screened prior to entry and provided with orientation and other supports, their performance on the post-residency certification examination was significantly lower than that of Canadian and American trained residents, with only slightly more than half passing the certification examination. The authors suggest a number of reasons for the IMGs' poorer performance, including variability of their undergraduate training, how and when they have learned to integrate their knowledge with clinical decision making, and the diversity of IMGs as a group.

On November 16, 2010, the Human Rights Tribunal released a report into allegations of discrimination against IMGs in Quebec. The findings of the report stated that foreign-trained doctors are subject to discriminatory treatment on the basis of their ethnic origin in the course of the admission process leading to postgraduate training in Quebec.

In response to this report, the Ontario Ministry of Health And Long Term Care commissioned an independent review of access to postgraduate programs by IMGs in Ontario. Judge Thomson produced an extensive report (Thomson & Cohl, 2011) addressing the analysis and background as well as findings and recommendations to make the process of admission of IMGs to postgraduate programs fair and transparent. Some of the recommendations from the Thomson Report were for research about predictors for success for IMGs on certification exams as well as research into admissions practices. In response to the Thomson report, the Thomson working group was struck to address these recommendations. A study looking at IMG admission data as predictors for success on college exams has been published (Schabort et al., 2014) and another to analyse this data for all programs in Ontario has been completed (Grierson et al., 2017). Another study looking at selection practices of IMGs and CMGs in Ontario is in progress.

Recent initiatives such as the Future of Medical Education in Canada (Best Practices in Applications and Selection Working Group, 2013) and the Thomson Report (Thomson & Cohl, 2011) have drawn attention to the process by which residency programs assess and select applicants (including IMGs) to their programs with particular attention to training the right mix of physicians to serve population health needs. In addition, there has recently been a substantial amount of interest in the literature around the psychometric properties of assessment tools. This report outlines the review process and the subsequent recommendations set forward by the Best Practices in Applications and Selection (BPAS) Working Group (2013), which consists of 13 principles and 20 best practices (Best Practices in Applications and Selection Working Group, 2013).

Based on the literature review and key informant interviews Walsh and colleagues (2011) have identified three key messages related to the successful training and certification of IMGs:

1. IMGs need orientation to provide them with the knowledge, both overt and tacit, required to integrate into the clinical and educational environment, as well as support programs for them and their families.
2. There is great diversity in the IMGs who come to Canada, which requires in depth assessment, both for proper placement and to allow postgraduate programs to adapt to their training needs. Resources are needed to meet this great diversity of learning needs.
3. Teachers need training to meet the specific needs of IMG residents.

Advice from IMGs for Future IMGs

I would like IMGs who are still thinking of applying to programs or give exams to be hopeful and confident as, irrespective of the number of failures, they may hear from friends, there are numerous successful stories as well. The only tip for IMGs to apply in Canada is to spend some time in the system, observing even if only for 1–2 weeks, and understanding the process of interviews, and above all, find another IMG who has done the program. As a female IMG, work life balance is difficult in the beginning but everything falls in place and truly Canadians at work and around are helpful and lovely people to be with. I would like to thank some of the mentors who themselves were IMGs who guided me through this process. I have met the most amazing people since being here and I am glad I made the decision to come here and not listen to all the negative discouraging stories that we hear most of the time when we contemplate beginning this process. (IMG narrative, fluidsurvey)

My final message to IMGs: do not give up, as long as you keep trying, you are going to get there. There is always light at the end of the tunnel. (IMG narrative, fluidsurvey)

Study hard, be hopeful and don't give up. (Malau-Aduli, 2011)

Speak loudly, clearly and confidently, and maintain good eye contact as that is the culture here, unlike back home where you are not allowed to question your lecturers' opinions or even make eye contacts with them. (Malau-Aduli, 2011)

The Ethics of Medical Migration

A final thought: Starfield and Fryer (2007) raised the very valid ethical dilemma of the United States disproportionately using graduates of foreign medical schools from the poorest and most deprived countries to maintain its primary care physician supply: "The ethical aspects of depending on foreign medical graduates is an important issue, especially when it deprives disadvantaged countries of their graduates to buttress a declining US primary care physician supply" (p. 486). How do we respond to this dilemma in Canada?

ACKNOWLEDGMENT

I would like to thank Dawn Elston, research coordinator, Department of Family Medicine McMaster University, for setting up fluidsurvey and conducting a content analysis whereby we compared women's narratives with predominant themes described in the literature narratives, and Alex Rewegaan, who did a literature search and retrieval and worked with Dawn on identifying themes in the fluidsurvey narratives.

REFERENCES

Association of Faculties of Medicine of Canada. (2006). AFMC modules 2006 IMGs. Retrieved from https://afmc.ca/timg/pdf/Intro_en.pdf

Association of Faculties of Medicine of Canada. (2009). Canadian medical education statistics. Retrieved from https://www.afmc.ca/pdf/cmes/CMES2009.pdf

Banner, S., & Comeau, M. (2006). Analysis of the 2006 survey of Canadians studying medicine and the medical schools training Canadians outside of Canada and the U.S. Final report to Health Canada. Ottawa: Health Canada.

Barry, James Miranda Stuart. (2008). In *The Canadian encyclopedia*. Retrieved from http://www.thecanadianencyclopedia.ca/en/m/article/james-barry/

Best Practices in Applications and Selection Working Group. (2013). *Best practices in applications and selection: Final report*. Toronto: University of Toronto Postgraduate Medical Education. Retrieved from http://pg.postmd.utoronto.ca/?ddownload=3919

Brandon, S. (2018). Barry, James (c.1799–1865). In *Oxford dictionary of national biography*. https://doi.org/10.1093/ref:odnb/1563

Broten, L. (2008). *Report on removing barriers for international medical doctors*. Ottawa: Minister of Health and Long-Term Care. Retrieved from http://www.health.gov.on.ca/en/common/ministry/publications/reports/removing_barriers/removing_barriers.aspx

Canadian Institute for Health Information. (2010). *Supply, distribution and migration of Canadian physicians, 2008*. Ottawa: CIHI. Retrieved from https://secure.cihi.ca/free_products/SMDB_2009_EN.pdf

Canadian Post-MD Education Registry. (2012). The national IMG database report. Retrieved from https://caper.ca/~assets/documents/2012_CAPER_National_IMG_Database_Report.pdf

Canadian Post-MD Education Registry. (2013). *2013–2014 annual census of post-MD trainees*. Retrieved from https://caper.ca/~assets/documents/pdf_2013-14_CAPER_Census.pdf

Canadian Resident Matching Service. (2010a). *Canadian medical graduate cohort data*. Retrieved from https://www.carms.ca/en/data-and-reports/r-1/reports-2010/

Canadian Resident Matching Service. (2010b). *Canadian students studying medicine abroad*. Ottawa: Author. Retrieved from http://www.carms.ca/pdfs/2010_CSA_Report/CaRMS_2010_CSA_Report.pdf

Collier, R. (2010, May 18). Medical school admission targets urged for rural and low-income Canadians. *CMAJ*, *182*(8), E327–E328. https://doi.org/10.1503/cmaj.109-3227 Medline:20371649

Crutcher, R.A., Banner, S.R., Szafran, O., & Watanabe, M. (2003, Apr 29). Characteristics of international medical graduates who applied to the CaRMS 2002 match. *CMAJ*, *168*(9), 1119–23. Medline:12719314

Curran, V., Hollett, A., Hann, S., & Bradbury, C. (2008, Autumn). A qualitative study of the international medical graduate and the orientation process. *Canadian Journal of Rural Medicine: The Official Journal of the Society of Rural Physicians of Canada*, *13*(4), 163–9. Medline:18845068

Dorgan, K.A., Lang, F., Floyd, M., & Kemp, E. (2009, Nov). International medical graduate-patient communication: a qualitative analysis of perceived barriers. *Academic Medicine: Journal of the Association of American Medical Colleges, 84*(11), 1567–75. https://doi.org/10.1097/ACM.0b013e3181baf5b1 Medline:19858820

du Preez, H.M. (2008, Jan). Dr James Barry: The early years revealed. *South African Medical Journal: Suid-Afrikaanse tydskrif vir geneeskunde, 98*(1), 52–8. Medline:18270643

du Preez, H.M. (2012). Dr James Barry (1789–1865): The Edinburgh years. *The Journal of the Royal College of Physicians of Edinburgh, 42*(3), 258–65. https://doi.org/10.4997/JRCPE.2012.315 Medline:22953323

Elkin, K., Spittal, M.J., & Studdert, D.M. (2012, Oct 15). Risks of complaints and adverse disciplinary findings against international medical graduates in Victoria and Western Australia. *The Medical Journal of Australia, 197*(8), 448–52. https://doi.org/10.5694/mja12.10632 Medline:23072241

Federal/Provincial/Territorial Advisory Committee on Health Delivery and Human Resources. (2004). *Report of the Canadian Task force on licensure of international medical graduates.* Ottawa: Health Canada.

Grierson, L.E.M., Mercuri, M., Brailovsky, C., Cole, G., Abrahams, C., Archibald, D., . . . Schabort, I. (2017). Admission factors associated with international medical graduate certification success: A collaborative retrospective review of postgraduate medical education programs in Ontario. *CMAJ, 5*(4), E785–90. http://doi.org/10.9778/cmajo.20170073

Hall, P., Keely, E., Dojeiji, S., Byszewski, A., & Marks, M. (2004, Mar). Communication skills, cultural challenges and individual support: challenges of international medical graduates in a Canadian healthcare environment. *Medical Teacher, 26*(2), 120–5. https://doi.org/10.1080/01421590310001653982 Medline:15203520

Harris, A. (2014). Encountering the familiar unknown: The hidden work of adjusting medical practice between local settings. *Journal of Contemporary Ethnography, 43*(3), 259–82. https://doi.org/10.1177/0891241613494810

Health Canada. (2003). Accord on health care renewal. Available at https://www.canada.ca/en/health-canada/services/health-care-system/health-care-system-delivery/federal-provincial-territorial-collaboration/2003-first-ministers-accord-health-care-renewal/2003-first-ministers-health-accord.html

Health Canada. (2004). The 2003 accord on health care renewal: A progress report. Retrieved from https://www.canada.ca/en/health-canada/services/health-care-system/health-care-system-delivery/federal-provincial-territorial-collaboration/first-ministers-meeting-year-plan-2004/2003-accord-health-care-renewal-progress.html

Huijskens, E.G., Hooshiaran, A., Scherpbier, A., & van der Horst, F. (2010, Aug). Barriers and facilitating factors in the professional careers of international medical graduates. *Medical Education, 44*(8), 795–804. https://doi.org/10.1111/j.1365-2923.2010.03706.x Medline:20633219

Kirby, M. (2002). *The health of Canadians – the federal role.* Report of the Standing Senate Committee on Social Affairs, Science and Technology. Retrieved from http://www.parl.gc.ca/37/2/parlbus/commbus/senate/com-e/soci-e/rep-e/repfinnov03-e.htm

Kubba, A.K. (2001). The life, work and gender of Dr James Barry MD (1795–1865). *Proceedings of the Royal College of Physicians of Edinburgh, 31*(4), 352–6. Medline:11833588

Leitch, R, (2001). The Barry room: The tale of a Pioneering military surgeon. Retrieved from https://web.archive.org/web/20070928030206/http://www.usmedicine.com/column.cfm?columnID=53&issueID=28

MacLellan, A.M., Brailovsky, C., Rainsberry, P., Bowmer, I., & Desrochers, M. (2010, Sep). Examination outcomes for international medical graduates pursuing or completing family medicine residency training in Quebec. *Canadian Family Physician Medecin de Famille Canadien, 56*(9), 912–18. Medline:20841596

Malau-Aduli, B.S. (2011, 06 25). Exploring the experiences and coping strategies of international medical students. *BMC Medical Education, 11*(1), 40–52. https://doi.org/10.1186/1472-6920-11-40 Medline:21702988

Merani, S., Abdulla, S., Kwong, J.C., Rosella, L., Streiner, D.L., Johnson, I.L., & Dhalla, I.A. (2010, Jun). Increasing tuition fees in a country with two different models of medical education. *Medical Education, 44*(6), 577–86. https://doi.org/10.1111/j.1365-2923.2010.03630.x Medline:20604854

Nightingale, F. (n.d.). *Letter to Parthenope, Lady Verney (undated).* London: Wellcome Institute for the History of Medicine.

Papadakis, M.A., Arnold, G.K., Blank, L.L., Holmboe, E.S., & Lipner, R.S. (2008, Jun 3). Performance during internal medicine residency training and subsequent disciplinary action by state licensing boards. *Annals of Internal Medicine, 148*(11), 869–76. https://doi.org/10.7326/0003-4819-148-11-200806030-00009 Medline:18519932

Pilotto, L.S., Duncan, G.F., & Anderson-Wurf, J. (2007, Aug 20). Issues for clinicians training international medical graduates: a systematic review. *The Medical Journal of Australia, 187*(4), 225–8. Medline:17708725

Romanow Commission. (2002). *Building on values: The future of health care in Canada—final report.* Retrieved from http://publications.gc.ca/collections/Collection/CP32-85-2002E.pdf

Schabort, I., Mercuri, M., & Grierson, L.E. (2014, Oct). Predicting international medical graduate success on college certification examinations: Responding to the Thomson and Cohl judicial report on IMG selection. *Canadian Family Physician Medecin de Famille Canadien, 60*(10), e478–e484. Medline:25316762

Sockalingam, S., Khan, A., Tan, A., Hawa, R., Abbey, S., Jackson, T., …, & Okrainec, A. (2014). A framework for understanding international medical graduate challenges during transition into fellowship programs. *Teaching and Learning in Medicine, 26*(4), 401–8. https://doi.org/10.1080/10401334.2014.945393 Medline:25318037

Starfield, B., & Fryer, G.E., Jr. (2007, Nov-Dec). The primary care physician workforce: ethical and policy implications. *Annals of Family Medicine, 5*(6), 486–91. https://doi.org/10.1370/afm.720 Medline:18025485

Szafran, O., Crutcher, R.A., Banner, S.R., & Watanabe, M. (2005, Sep). Canadian and immigrant international medical graduates. *Canadian Family Physician Medecin de Famille Canadien, 51*, 1242–3. Medline:16926941

Tamblyn, R., Abrahamowicz, M., Dauphinee, D., Wenghofer, E., Jacques, A., Klass, D., …, & Hanley, J.A. (2007, Sep 5). Physician scores on a national clinical skills examination as predictors of complaints to medical regulatory authorities. *JAMA, 298*(9), 993–1001. https://doi.org/10.1001/jama.298.9.993 Medline:17785644

Tamblyn, R., Abrahamowicz, M., Dauphinee, W.D., Hanley, J.A., Norcini, J., Girard, N., …, & Brailovsky, C. (2002, Dec 18). Association between licensure examination scores and practice in primary care. *JAMA, 288*(23), 3019–26. https://doi.org/10.1001/jama.288.23.3019 Medline:12479767

Terry, D.R., Lê, Q., & Hoang, H. (2014, 12 31). Satisfaction amid professional challenges: International medical graduates in rural Tasmania. *The Australasian Medical Journal, 7*(12), 500–17. https://doi.org/10.4066/AMJ.2014.2267 Medline:25646126

Thind, A., Freeman, T., Cohen, I., Thorpe, C., Burt, A., & Stewart, M. (2007, Aug). Characteristics and practice patterns of international medical graduates: How different are they from those of Canadian-trained physicians? *Canadian Family Physician, 53*(8), 1330–1. Medline:17872850

Thomson, G., & Cohl, K. (2011). *IMG selection: Independent review of access to postgraduate programs by international medical graduates in Ontario*. Retrieved from http://www.health.gov.on.ca/en/common/ministry/publications/reports/thomson/v1_thomson.pdf

Walsh, A., Banner, S., Schabort, I., Armson, H., Bowmer, I., & Granata, B. (2011). *International medical graduates—Current issues*. Ottawa: Future of

Medical Education in Canada Postgraduate. Retrieved from https://afmc.ca/pdf/fmec/05_Walsh_IMG%20Current%20Issues.pdf
Wong, A., & Lohfeld, L. (2008, Jan). Recertifying as a doctor in Canada: international medical graduates and the journey from entry to adaptation. *Medical Education*, *42*(1), 53–60. https://doi.org/10.1111/j.1365-2923.2007.02903.x Medline:18086199

SECTION THREE

Career Experience: Examining Cultural Patterns within the Medical Community and Health Care System

Despite medicine's cultural proclivity to regard being a physician as a genderless profession, there is ample evidence that women's experience within the profession differs from that of their male counterparts. There are distinct challenges for women physicians in sharing their stories – and for researchers seeking to examine the differences between how men and women experience the culture of medicine and of being a physician. Having a different narrative as a woman is often dismissed by those who insist the practice of medicine from the physician standpoint is gender-neutral; attempting to defend the different experiences of women physicians is often seen as sexist, perpetuating a perspective that female physicians are "less" than male physicians.

The two chapters in this section present distinct perspectives on the cultural patterns of medicine: in Chapter 7, Kathleen Gartke and Janet Dollin present an academic approach to exploring the different influences, factors, and issues in the career trajectories of female physicians. In Chapter 8, Shelley Ross (a late-career female physician) shares a very personal perspective on her career trajectory, presenting both the advantages and the disadvantages she perceived in navigating a medical career that included advocacy and leadership.

7 Career Trajectory of Women in Medicine: Taming the Winds That Blow Us

KATHLEEN GARTKE AND JANET DOLLIN

Introduction

The career trajectory of women in medicine is often described as nonlinear. This chapter will discuss the various vectors and forces that shape the path throughout a woman's life cycle. Women in medicine, out of biological necessity as much as out of maximizing personal strengths, have led the way to renewed efforts at harmonizing employment with personal life. They have led the way in naming and taming the barriers to their advancement. The workforce is better off for these efforts: better off because there is strength in diversity and better off because these are human values and not simply gendered ones. Naming the barriers is a necessary first step in creating systemic change; taming them will require more.

Systems Issues from a Life Cycle Perspective: Choosing a Career in Medicine

Choosing a career in medicine has been an adventure chosen by more women than men for some time. This demographic tidal wave began in 1995, when women first made up more than half of medical students. Canadian medical school classes in 2013–14 were 55.9% female and have been greater than 55% for over 10 years (Association of Faculties of Medicine of Canada [AFMC], 2014). Women in medicine have entered what has been, in the past, a male-only profession. Indeed, the barriers to entry into medical school were very real to the current female faculty teaching this year's medical student population, most of whom have no such personal memory. The 1970 graduating class had 15.7%

women, that of 1980 had 36%, while 1990 had 44%. This demographic shift has been accompanied by evolution in the profession of medicine. With their influx into medicine, women have been perceived as agents of some of this change, as better listeners with a different communication style (Phillips, 2013). Medicine has transitioned from a paternalistic style of practice to one that is more collaborative. By virtue of the many women patients who preferentially choose to see female physicians, the practices of the latter have swelled with female patients, thus making them experts in the growing field of women's health. By virtue of the biological necessity, moving female physicians into and out of the workforce has brought much change in work patterns and options, with more flexibility now available to all practitioners.

Choosing a career in medicine, however, was not always a possibility for women. Women in Canada were banned from attending medical schools until the admittance of Augusta Stowe-Gullen to the University of Toronto, from which she graduated in 1883, becoming the first woman to do so in Canada. Her mother, Emily Stowe, was the first woman to practice medicine in Canada in 1868, but she had received her degree in the United States. Emily is credited with founding the Women's Medical College in Toronto (Dollin, 2002).

When she graduated high school in 1885, Maude Abbott was awarded a scholarship to attend McGill University. Her dream of higher education had become possible thanks to an endowment given to McGill the year before. She subsequently hit the glass ceiling of her day upon graduating with her BA in 1900. With the University of Toronto's medical school policy as a background, the campaign to admit women into the faculty of medicine at McGill was started by the "radical" behaviour of a classmate named Grace Ritchie, who was two years ahead of Maude. Ritchie courageously defied authority by surreptitiously inserting statements previously censored by the principal of McGill into her valedictory speech of 1887. Courageous for her era, but considered disgraceful, she was ostracized for the attempt and left town for better climates (in her case, Kingston), unknowingly paving the way for Maude to continue the campaign. Maude's 1889 request for admission to medical school was quickly refused – "let other universities lower their standards if they want to" (Knoeff & Zwijnenberg, 2015, p. 58).

Maude ultimately attended Bishop's University, fighting from there for clerkship positions at the McGill hospitals. However, she left that chilly climate for Vienna, to study at what was the Mecca for her interests in pathology. When she returned to Montreal, she was expected to drop all the expertise she had gained to care for women and children, as was expected of women doctors of her day. Instead she accepted an offer at McGill as curator of the museum of medical anatomy, going on to publish her own textbook of anatomical pathology and ultimately contributing to Osler's text, *System of Medicine*, published in 1908. McGill had to take notice, granting her an honorary MDCM degree in 1910. Some 14 years later, McGill agreed to accept women into its medical school, and Maude Abbott became a founding member of the Federation of Medical Women of Canada. This organization, still active today, advocates for the well-being and advancement of women physicians. Maude Abbott was the ultimate example of the "just do it" approach – not really as a vocal activist for women in medicine, but rather an example of high achievement that was impossible to ignore.

Cultural Climate Issues in Medicine

> Placing women on political equality with men would cause domestic strife … The majority of women are emotional, and if given the franchise would be a menace rather than an aid.
>
> – Manitoba Premier Sir Rodmond Roblin 1914

Interestingly, this 1914 quote speaks to an attitude that in 100 years has certainly evolved but has not completely disappeared. Despite so many remarkable advances towards equity in this century, it still cannot be said that women have fully arrived. Women are not evenly represented across all specialties, nor have they penetrated all levels of leadership in proportion to their numbers at entry levels. What factors contribute to this reality? Societal expectations of women? Do women have free choice, or does the still-male-dominated environment direct them into career paths while denying them a place at the highest levels of leadership? While there are no definitive answers, there are a number of research studies looking at the climate in medical education.

The "chilly climate," a phrase coined in 1969 by academic Dr Bernice Sandler (Sandler et al., 1996), creates an educational environment that is filled with subtle and subliminal messages, an environment that is less than welcoming to women students and is especially discouraging to those who choose to push traditional female boundaries. Harassment and intimidation, based on gender, continue to contribute to this chilly climate. Hazing, sexist jokes, and the so-called rape culture are sadly still a reality in universities today. The Internet has added a new dimension to sexual harassment. In 2014 a Facebook group of male dental students at Dalhousie University posted rude, misogynistic, and sexist comments about their female classmates. Reaction to this poisoned virtual environment was strong, and discussions around how to deal with the perpetrators raged for months. Unfortunately, privacy considerations meant that any final consequences for these men, remain confidential. Sexist jokes in real life were the first to be named and shamed. On line, however, sexist jokes are freely posted and easily found. Social media is where most of our newest generation of professional students live and communicate, and represent a new space defining the climate of a medical school. These sexist postings were a revelation for this professional school, where sexism was believed no longer to exist. Women still experience virtual and overt sexism, although this varies across different cultures and environments. There does appear to be an improvement with time and with education, although the true efficacy of these measures has been questioned. Harder still to comprehend is how forcefully a society's ingrained gender-discriminatory attitudes can manifest, even when they are believed to have been resolved. In 2017 and 2018 we finally saw the clear, new calling out of previously hidden yet overt sexual abuse, harassment, and intimidation with the#MeTooInMedicine movement.

Microaggressions are defined as "everyday verbal, non-verbal and environmental slights, snubs or insults – whether intentional or unintentional – that communicate hostile, derogatory or negative messages to targets, based solely upon their membership in a marginalized group" (Wing Sue, 2010). These micro inequities, subtle differences in how our men and women are treated, are harder to address, but ultimately do not allow them to benefit from the full spectrum of human capacity. These powerful winds blow men and women into gendered career paths beginning well before undergraduate education and extending to postgraduate and faculty levels. Fewer opportunities and more obstacles are reported in medicine and in all academic sciences (Settles et al., 2006).

In a 2012 study rating hireability of applicants for a laboratory manager job, researchers found that the exact same curriculum vitae, when attributed to a male, led to higher ratings of competence and greater hireability, as well as to recommendations for higher starting salaries and more research support. This was true whether the assessor of the CV was male or female. When the CV was attributed to a woman, both male and female faculty found her more likeable than when they believed they were assessing a man. Stereotypes of women and men influence everyone subconsciously while impacting women in negative ways (Moss-Racusina et al., 2012).

Women are still expected to fulfil gendered roles in the family and in the classroom, laboratory, or clinic. Despite large increases in the numbers of women medical students, harassment and gender stereotyping continue to detract from their education and opportunities (Bickel, 2001).

Generational Differences

Jolly et al. (2014) found that high-achieving Generation X males continued to perform less domestic work than women. Women were more likely to take time off after children arrived and were more likely to report that family obligations impeded work achievement. Men with a part-time employed or unemployed spouse had difficulty understanding this problem. Female physicians were more likely to have a spouse who is employed full time, and "men attempt to preserve some presentation of themselves as masculine and because domestic labour is culturally defined as feminine, not doing it is masculine" (Jolly et al., 2014, p. 351). These researchers go on to suggest that many women and men remain committed, whether behaviourally or ideologically, to an unequal division of domestic labour. These concepts of domestic division of labour will likely change over time because of changes in the belief systems of the newer generations of physicians.

A generation is a group of people whose characteristics were shaped and defined by the societal events that occurred during their formative years. Not every member of a particular generation will share everything in common with other members of that generation, so these concepts are stereotypes and not always followed.

Traditionalists, Veterans, or the "Silent Generation" were born 1930–1945. Baby boomers, the "sandwich" generation, were born from 1946 to 1964, and these individuals are now the older faculty members. Generation X, "baby busters," who were born from 1965 to 1976, are mid- or early level faculty and have the strongest leadership potential at this time. Generation Y or "millennials" who were born from 1977 to 1991 are the residents and early faculty. Generation Z, "new millennials," born 1991 or later, are the happiest and most technology-savvy current students. Generational differences in attitudes, behaviours, expectations, motivations, and communication styles are seen to create miscommunication between generations (Psychology Foundation, n.d.).

Baby boomers prize ambition, invention, and hard work, and demand respect based on expertise and accomplishment. They are a group deeply invested in their profession as a major part of their identity. They demand respect but still demonstrate some gender bias. Boomers, the last generation to have used typewriters, will shortly create a major demographic shift or brain drain as they all reach the point of retirement.

Generation X, a fun-loving, self-reliant, somewhat troubled, cynical, misunderstood group have a narrowing gender gap and consider themselves gender-neutral. They prize diversity, balance, free time, and prefer to work to live. Perhaps they feel that what were gender barriers in the past are now more broad-based (Cochran et al., 2013). Gen Xers, some having witnessed the burnouts of their parents, have a better work-life balance than their boomer parents. Retaining them requires flexible and efficient workplaces, so that more time can be spent with family.

The Generation Y millennials are family-oriented, mobile, consumerist, brand conscious, hopeful, idealistic, and the most gender neutral. With a population base three times as big as Gen X, they demand flexibility and work-life balance, and prize individuality – qualities not typical of traditional surgical specialty training (Dageforde et al., 2013). They are marrying earlier again and having children when younger. They prize values of tolerance, cooperation, connection, and communication. Expert understanding of emerging technology has allowed them to feel constantly in contact with friends and family. Expectations for work-life balance from this large cohort will likely translate into decreased hours worked by physicians of both sexes and more demand for less than full-time work and job flexibility.

Generation Z, or new millennials, are the youngest group in the workforce now. Extremely techno-savvy, they prefer instant messaging and feel email is for "old folks." Confident, happy, and secure, they are team players, and like to engage in community service activities. They are gender-blind global citizens with unprecedented activism who work well in teams and value volunteerism, showing a renewed sense of civic responsibility. It remains to be seen what impact they will have on work-life balance. An awareness of differing needs and expectations by generational cohorts is important in the untangling of any gender differences.

Choosing a Medical Discipline

- The role of chance, of mentors, and of change

The National Physician Survey (2014a) shows that in 2014, 61% of the global physician workforce in Canada was male, while 39% was female. This is not evenly reflected within specialties. Currently, the specialist workforce is male dominated at 66%, with 34% being female, while the family medicine workforce is closer to parity at 56% male and 44% female (National Physician Survey, 2014a) The literature is filled with articles describing gendered choices in medical specialty training. For example, surgery is predominantly preferred by men, and gynecology, pediatrics, and family practice by women. Factors that influence these choices are personal values around child care, personal support systems such as expectations of equality at home, spousal career dominance, or having a spouse who will share family requirements (Alers et al., 2014). Individual aspects such as personal ambition, future perspective, and work-life balance were found to be more important than occupational aspects such as job variety or job-related ambition. Perceived family compatibility improves certain specialties as a choice for women more so than men (Kiolbassa et al., 2011).

Family medicine is the most common career choice for women in medicine. Phillips (2013) reports that women practice differently than men. They see fewer patients, spend more time per patient, and address prevention more often. Communication and patient satisfaction are more highly valued by women practitioners. Overall, their hours worked may be fewer. Measures of patient wellness or measures of patient preference may be of more importance, and new ways of addressing population health other than measuring the number of physicians per population unit or the number of patient visits per physician may be needed. These factors must be addressed in both their positive and their negative impacts on our health human resources (Phillips, 2013).

Where and when a student trains will create an influential environment around the student. Perceptions or experience of a lack of work-life balance was the most common reason for women to reject specific specialty choices of surgery, emergency medicine, or certain hospital-based specialties (Goldacre et al., 2012).

The presence or absence of role models living the life of happy and balanced clinicians matters to the trainee. Dyrbye and colleagues (2012) found that 52.5% of a surgical workforce had experienced work-life conflict in the three weeks before their study, which correlated to a higher risk for depression, burnout, and alcohol abuse. There was also a lower chance these surgeons would recommend a surgical specialty to their own children, let alone be good role models to trainees. These surgeons were more likely to be planning to reduce hours worked or leave practice, leading to human resource issues from both their absence and the drop in trainees attracted to this program (Dyrbye et al., 2012).

Men and women experience each rotation they do differently. Where negative or positive role models exist, students' choices are influenced. The climate of a specialty is vital. Some specialties prize masculine traits like strength, decisiveness, action orientation (e.g., surgery), while some prize feminine ones such as nurturing, communication, and collaboration (e.g., pediatrics). As more women enter family medicine, the question becomes how our male students will learn specific skills when patients request female physicians, or how female students will learn specific skills when surgical paradigms may exclude them.

Hill and Giles (2014) argue that gender (rather than biological sex) is a learned behaviour and discursive constraints, such as gender, social class, ethnicity, and sexuality, restrict available choices. We are a product of our backgrounds (personal and social), and we only have the illusion of choice (Hill & Giles, 2014).

Choosing Academics or Not

- Work life policies: flexible jobs, job sharing, stop the clock
- Parental leaves
- Child care choices

Academic medicine needs better benefit from the demographic shift towards more women. The 2011–12 GWIMS benchmarking report shows that in the United States, women make up 20% of professors, 14% of department chairs, and 13% of medical school deans. Explanations focus on choice (career decisions and preferences) or constraint (e.g., discrimination and implicit bias) or some complex interrelationship between the two (Association of American Medical Colleges, 2013).

Career choice or inequitable climate are discussed by Zhuge et al. (2011) who report similarly discrepant figures for women in academic leadership worldwide. This global disparity is attributed to the sticky floor of micro inequities and a leaky pipeline of women being less likely to be promoted, even when adjusted for number of publications, amount of grants, hours worked, specialty, or career track. When all else is equal, women are less likely to be asked to serve in leadership roles. Pay for full female professors, when all else is equal, lags behind that of their male counterparts by $12,777 to $23,764. The researchers discuss three major constraints: traditional gender roles, manifestations of sexism in the medical environment, and a dearth of effective mentors (Zhuge et al., 2011).

Medical students are older now than they were in the past and must make decisions about their medical discipline exactly when their own biological clocks are starting to tick louder. The members of their generational cohort have different values than in the past. Having accomplished undergraduate degrees before medical school, these older students are making key career decisions at a difficult time.

Academic medicine is a rewarding, high-powered career option. Benchmarking shows the inequities that exist. The nature of academic medicine has been changing as women enter and advance and begin to notice the need to fight for work-life balance, flexible jobs, job sharing, stop-the-clock policies, parental leaves, and childcare choices.

Career Advancement, However You Define It

- What counts for promotion?
- What makes a leader?

Women must do more than men to be considered competent or equal. Papers, artworks, and CVs thought to be women's rated less highly than those thought to be men's. Grants submitted with women's names must get higher scores to be funded. Women faculty must smile more and be more nurturing than men faculty to receive equal ratings (Valarian, 1998). As well, women have hit their own psychological glass ceiling as a consequence of having lived in their personal social environments with their inherent influences, according to Austin (2001), a psychiatrist.

What counts for promotion is as important as who feels they should count for promotion. Women are less likely to advance themselves, less likely to see their work as important, and less likely to be tapped for promotion or awards by colleagues. Without being conscious of their mental models of gender, both men and women devalue women's work and allow women a narrower band of assertive behaviour. Women face many more challenges than men in obtaining career-advancing mentoring. Isolation reduces women's capacity for risk-taking, often translating into either a reluctance to pursue professional goals or a protective response, such as perfectionism.

Despite increased numbers of women, there has not been a parallel increase in publications by women authoring original articles in traditional major journals. Women are also not invited as authors of guest editorials in proportion to their numbers. This will not change until there are more senior women. For women to become senior, there will need to be more publications by women, a vicious circle not lost on the policy front (Hamel et al., 2006).

There is more awareness of alternative styles of research, with women doing more qualitative research, hence publishing in non-traditional journals or reporting to "alternative" publications. Women's work as teachers, or on committees that guide policy, or even one-on-one coaching or mentoring work may not count as visible promotion criteria. Women lead differently, and expecting them to advance in traditional ways will fail. Eagly et al. (2003) describe "transformational" leaders who inspire followers' commitment and creativity, and "transactional" leaders who appeal to subordinates' self-interest using reward and punishment as incentives ("command and control"). Women are more likely than men to use transformational style. Women are more likely to advance in flatter, more matrixed organizations than in hierarchical ones (Eagly et al., 2003).

Women are more likely to use constellations of behaviours that are communal, such as niceness, sympathy, friendliness, and gentleness, while men are more likely to lead with agency: more aggressiveness, ambition, self-confidence, dominance, forcefulness, self-reliance, and individualism. These qualities are found to different degrees in both men and women (Dollin, 2016). The roles given, as well as the expectations of others, influence the degree to which these various skills are used. Gender bias creates an expectation of communal behaviours from women. "Niceness" becomes a norm and is less likely to be valued as highly as boldness and charisma when promotion is considered. Aggression becomes unexpected, and for the woman, derogatory descriptors like "pushy" replace what for a man would be called "strong" (Heim, 2001).

Physician Health Issues

> A blank wall of social and professional antagonism faces the woman physician that forms a situation of singular and painful loneliness, leaving her without support, respect, or professional counsel.
>
> – Elizabeth Blackwell

Childbearing

There is a biological imperative for women in medicine. Childbearing, if that is a choice a young physician wants to make, must be timed to occur during ideal fertility years. In addition, students' increasingly long premedical education has led to an older cohort of students who reach that biological imperative point earlier in their training. That said, children are identified as the most important obstacle on the way to the top of a medical career (Kuehn, 2012). Negative bias persists for women who choose pregnancy while in training. This negative bias is greater among male colleagues and faculty, but a significant number of females also hold negative views; more than half of surgical candidates delay pregnancy until after training (Turner et al., 2012).

Choosing to have children or not comes up at key educational times for women in medicine, coinciding with key service requirements. Women in fields such as medicine and law have had lower marriage rates, higher likelihood of being childless, and fewer children than the national average. Women who hold graduate and professional degrees end their childbearing years with 1.6 children, compared with 2.4 children for women without such degrees, and they are more often childless than those who end formal education with graduation from high school (Turner et al., 2012, p. 478). There are many reasons for this, but as more women in medicine are seen, it is anticipated that some of the barriers to childbearing that existed in the past will improve with time and appropriate intervention (Turner et al., 2012).

More women are going into surgery since an 80-hour cap on the workweek was established in the United States in 2003. Learning and service environments have not been friendly to pregnancy. Announcing a pregnancy inevitably leads to negative reactions from colleagues who are thinking about call schedules. Compared to 30 years ago, more women surgeons now have a pregnancy during their training (63.1% in the past decade versus 38.5% 30 years ago; Kuehn, 2012). In a survey of women surgeons, it was found that while women in this field choose to have their babies significantly later than the US norms, they do indeed have them – it might be better to plan for this rather than be annoyed about it (Kuehn, 2012).

Waiting for the right time to have babies will lead to increased age and decreased fertility (Miura & Boxer, 2013). Overall pregnancy complication rates were increased (31% versus 14%) in this study group compared to matched women in the general population. For those working over 60 hours per week, there was an association with preterm babies. Residents subsequently took shorter maternity leaves and breastfed for shorter periods. Female residents in internal medicine, pediatrics, and surgery are less likely to plan to have children during residency than male counterparts (27% versus 41%) (Hamilton et al., 2012). Delaying childbearing, however, has inherent risks of missing the window of peak fertility, and the subsequent risks and complications of decreased fertility, new reproductive technologies, and multiple births.

Mid-Career

Medicine has the capacity to be an incredibly flexible and rewarding profession. A career can be varied and take different shapes at different points in a physician's life. A woman may decide to work less than full time at one point and then ramp it up at another. Off ramps, on ramps, and speed bumps exist and should be considered. Where men's careers are described as linear, continually moving upwards, women's tend to be nonlinear, at times circular, and are well described by Anne Seiden (1989) as "life pretzels."

Overwork is a common problem within medicine in general. Traditionally success and busy-ness were intertwined. Medicine was a calling and little was said about balance. Hours were grueling and were seen as an initiation rite or a badge of courage. Perhaps with the increase of women in medicine, perhaps with a generational ideological shift, perhaps related to an aging workforce who also reduce work hours (Sarma et al., 2011), life and expectation of work hours has thankfully changed. Burnout, depression, and exhaustion are key mid-career problems, and this is a welcome shift in preventing them.

According to the National Physician Survey (2014b) women without dependents worked 52 hours per week compared to men at 53 hours – both significantly over the national average for workers in most other jobs. With children under five, this changes to 42 hours for women versus 55 hours for men; with children ages 5 to 10, it is 46 hours for women and 58 hours for men, and with children over 10, it is 47 versus 52 hours. Is this really part time? Is guilt over not contributing or blame for lack of commitment necessary? To say women work fewer hours is only a relative term. Relative to a time when overwork was the norm? Relative to a time when men played a less time-involved role in caregiving for their families? Relative to other Canadians? Being married and having children results in women working fewer hours. Clearly working fewer hours will have a human health resource impact, but if work-life balance is to be increasingly valued by all, this is an issue to thank women in medicine for raising. This issue needs to be solved for the sake of the health of both men and women.

At mid-career, women see childrearing as an addition to the many other demands of an active career. Women pressure themselves to be more efficient, tend to be perfectionist, and are reticent to see themselves as leaders or to apply for top positions. Early recognition of overload, work-life conflicts, and overstress should prevent "burnout or boreout" (Schueller-Weidekamm & Kautzky-Willer, 2012, p. 249). This recognition is essential to prevent the high substance abuse and suicide rates for both men and women in medicine. Women physicians are three to four times as likely and men 1.5 times as likely to attempt suicide as the population averages (Shrier & Shrier, 2009).

Duxbury and Higgins (2003) found that women in this "full nest" stage of mid-career devote more hours per week than men to non-work activities, such as child care and eldercare, and are more likely to have primary responsibility for non-work tasks. In their landmark study, 70% of respondents were parents (average number of children for parents in the sample is 2.1); 60% had eldercare responsibilities (average number of elderly dependants is 2.3); 13% had responsibility for the care of a disabled relative; and 13% had both child care and eldercare demands. Women were more likely than men to report high levels of role overload and high caregiver strain. These work-life strains were associated with more mental health problems and absenteeism. They were associated with poor recruitment and retention, and, importantly, with poor family outcomes, leaving these women less able to enjoy and nurture their families. The ultimate impact on Canadian families is at stake here. The authors conclude that their findings support the research literature in the area, which suggests that the role of working mother is qualitatively different from the role of working father, and that the "quality" of motherhood as a role is not as high as fatherhood (i.e., dads do the fun family tasks while mothers do the hard stuff). They go on to suggest that it is not known if these differences are due to social, workplace, or family factors (or some combination) and recommend more research so that targeted policies may be developed and supports implemented. More equitable sharing of child rearing within the family may lead to better mental health outcomes for working mothers, they suggest (Duxbury & Higgins, 2003).

It is women who choose to define their own paths by working less than full time in community and not academic settings, with less prestigious specialties, fewer leadership positions and fewer mentors, yet most interestingly they are the women who define themselves as most satisfied with their careers overall (Buddeberg-Fischer et al., 2010).

It is also at mid-career that decisions are seen to change paths altogether. One qualitative study looked at the factors that lead academic women to choose to leave that path. Key factors were (1) a lack of role models in combining work and family, (2) frustration with research (funding, mentorship, competition), (3) work-life imbalance, and (4) negative institutional environment (non-collaborative and biased towards males). These women reviewed their priorities and decided that theirs did not match those of their institution, which led to them being undervalued (Levine et al., 2011). A higher percentage of women than men agreed that different factors are obstacles, such as meetings after 5 p.m. and on weekends, rigid promotion timelines, no emergency child care, no part-time tenure track, no formal parental leave policy, and no onsite child care. Even poor quality of sleep on work days had a greater influence in pushing women to leave than it did for men (Estryn-Behar et al., 2011).

Late Career

- Aging workforce and aging population

Exiting careers for leave, then re-entering, and then re-exiting for caregiving roles are facts for many women physicians. There are few services or supports geared specifically to these necessities. Both men and women would benefit from improved workplace flexibility, job sharing, and family friendliness within medicine. Like the early and mid-career phases, the late careers of women in medicine are punctuated by the additional demands of a now-grown family and older parents. Female patterns of career trajectory remain twisted or nonlinear. Now there are issues of personal health, caregiving for family members, and the same issues of work-life balance. Perhaps when childrearing is over, women are more able to focus on their careers. Increasing population longevity suggests that women physicians will be taking care of parents for longer than in the past. Data on work hours, however, shows that all physicians, both male and female, tend to reduce hours worked after age 65.

The average age of physicians has remained relatively stable over the past five years (49.7 in 2009 and 50.3 in 2013). An increasing number of younger physicians entering the workforce may influence this trend (Canadian Institute for Health Information [CIHI], 2014).

This is not so for the Canadian population whose aging will seriously challenge the health system's capacity to care for them: 12% of family practitioners and 16% of specialists are 65 years old or older (National Physician Survey, 2014a). What these physicians will do as they wind down their careers will greatly influence health human resources. Canadian statistics suggest that it is women who are increasing indirect care while decreasing direct patient care (Sarma et al., 2011). Perhaps this is through more work in community health centres or alternative settings where there are teams of health providers, not all of whom are physicians. As this cohort ages, this group of baby boomers will not fully drop out of practice when they retire, but will likely reduce practice hours or practice scope, or be more involved in non-clinical work or in multidisciplinary teams. This will have implications in planning for medical human resource needs (CIHI, 2014).

The Practice of Medicine – Learning the Business

- Medical human resource planning and policies
- Leading change – for patients, for policy, for politics

> Forget conventionalisms; forget what the world will say, whether you are in or out of your place; think your best thoughts, speak your best words, do your best works, looking to your own conscience for approval.
>
> – Susan B. Anthony

It was the women's movement in the 1960s that noticed that the personal barriers for each individual woman were linked to the policies that define the world, and in this case, the workplace. "The personal is political" became the rallying cry. This is important to remember as policy is discussed, since each independent and strong woman doctor need not feel that she is discovering these barriers on her own when she reaches that point in her own career. The themes of the barriers to women's advancement are known, and solutions to the problems need to be addressed collectively as there will be more influence in numbers.

To address barriers, they must be named and defined. Benchmarking the current situation comes next, followed by the development of tools to measure success and, consequently, any policy needed to correct a historical path needing correction. Many groups have formed with the mission to be a collective voice for women in medicine, and many others are doing the necessary groundwork to be able to move things forward. What may have begun as informal networking groups for women in medicine have grown in depth and in number in response to many structured women in medicine (WIM) programs. The Federation of Medical Women of Canada (FMWC), which turns 100 in 2014, is committed to the professional, social, and personal advancement of women physicians and to the promotion of the well-being of women, both in the medical profession and in society at large. The American Medical Women's Association is a parallel group in the United States, and both are under the umbrella of the Medical Women's International Association. These organizations, and others, have been working to address the advancement of women in medicine, to name the inequities, to increase leadership, and to develop tools for monitoring and forward thinking policies. Some of these tools are available online for sharing, both validated (Westring et al., 2012) and invalidated (AFMC, 2010) ones. In Canada the Association of Faculties of Medicine of Canada (AFMC) has an equity, diversity, and gender committee, and each of the medical schools strives to have an officer or committee whose mandate is to address these issues locally and represent the school nationally. In the United States, the Association of American Medical Colleges (AAMC) has surveyed and given guidance to US medical schools. Other groups for women in medicine and science exist as well and references to their different benchmarking surveys and policy recommendations can be found in this chapter (Group for Women in Medicine and Science [GWIMS], World Organization of National Colleges, Academies and Academic Associations of General Practitioners/Family Physicians, and Working Party for Women in Family Medicine). Other non-female-only groups have contributed with focused programs for women, such as Executive Leadership in Academic Medicine and Society for Physician Executives. Non-medical women's groups such as Women's Executive Network or Women in STEM (science, technology, engineering, and math), or University Women, have all addressed these same issues as well. Thus, no one needs to feel alone in facing personal barriers, and the wheel does not need to be reinvented regarding the need to change policy.

One of the first barriers described for women in medicine was the dearth of female role models in leadership positions. This triggered the development of informal, and then formal mentoring programs. Mentors were seen as vital links in academic environments offering support for careers as well as for work-life balance. In a letter to the editor of *Academic Medicine*, Arora and Galanos (2011) highlight the importance of not settling for the progress made through having mentors but of continuing the effort. A mentor listens and gives guidance and encouragement. Understanding has evolved over time; sponsors are now also available who are more pro-active in opening doors, as well as coaches who help women build new behaviours to achieve their personal best and to lead policy change (Arora & Galanos, 2011).

Susan Phillips (2013) describes "the double bind" of women, who need to focus on family, being considered uncommitted to career, and vice versa. While this is clearly not true, attitudes do influence choices. This translates into work choices, which may ultimately disadvantage women. Awareness of how attitude shapes career choice and even policy is needed for collective action. Opening a practice is a foray into business taken by fewer women than men. Learning the ropes of hiring and firing are skills that are learnable but rarely taught. These skills have gendered nuances. Choosing to work less than full time in a clinical office will require collaboration with others and the formation of groups. Job sharing remains rare in medical or surgical residencies or within faculty positions, but clinic sharing is growing.

Provincial and territorial policy requirements also influence how one can juggle the various components of a career. In Quebec, for example, recently proposed changes to policy will require doctors to work specific numbers of hours in hospitals and long-term-care settings, in addition to offices where they will have to see specific volumes of patients. This will make working less than full time virtually impossible and will curtail women's control over their career path. Having a sense of autonomy or control over career choice is one of the major factors that prevent burnout.

Policy – One of the Winds That Buffet

Policy at all levels should help shape us but instead follows us, in so far as it tends to reflect our attitudes, values, desires and more practically speaking, our present situation. Does this lagging behind nature of policy make it an irrelevant tool for change? Probably not. Change across our society occurs at different speeds. Leaders, or those that recognize a new need, can identify problems and suggest solutions. After appropriate study of the results of new interventions, this information should become the feeding ground for policymakers. In this way, policy changes can pull the rest of the group up to speed and help develop a new platform for ongoing and progressive change.

The practice of medicine in Canada is directed by policies at multiple levels. Health care is considered a provincial or territorial matter, but is overseen at the federal level where transfer payments to the provinces and territories to pay for health care originate. Each has its own medical college that oversees physician licensing and discipline matters and has a Ministry of Health that negotiates or imposes fee schedules. The Royal College of Physicians and Surgeons of Canada oversees the certification of specialty practice as does the College of Family Physicians. Many physicians practise in an academic hospital setting, which may or may not be attached to a university. These hospitals and universities all have multiple policymaking bodies to which the physician/medical student is answerable, in addition to their licensing body, their certification body, and their Ministry of Health. Education is provincially or territorially directed, affecting medical students in all 17 Canadian medical schools. The ministries of health fund individual physicians as well as hospitals. Historically, physicians practised medicine following a "pay for service" model. Increasingly, alternative forms of payment have led to 50% of family physicians receiving remuneration from an alternative source (Sarma et al., 2011). This has put the physician into an employee role, adding employment policy/law from both the federal and provincial or territorial levels to the mix of policy that directs physicians, without the benefits normally accruing to employees. One hundred years of change in policy have helped to shape a gradual feminization of medicine. Early women in medicine were pioneers, dealing with associated issues and challenges with one-off solutions. By the 1970s, women made up only 25% or less of the students in Canadian medical schools. This number rose to almost 50% by the turn of the twenty-first century (2000), and in many cases is now much higher (up to 70%). At this point, all too often women still seek one-off answers in situations where policies to help them with career choices either do not yet exist or are not readily available. Discrimination based on gender is illegal in Canada – one example of a law that has followed societal change. It is hoped that closer examination of the subtle gender bias, which continues to exist, will help lead policy development and laws going forward.

While in the past, the decision to pursue a career in medicine was, for the most part, made at the secondary school level, the majority of schools now expect most candidates for medical education to have completed an undergraduate degree. Women currently make up the majority of these graduates of undergraduate education. In 2009 (US figures), women made up 57% of awarded bachelor degrees, 60% of masters, and 52% of doctoral degrees (Dageforde et al., 2013). This changes the demographics of the applicant pool. It is small wonder that medical school classes are greater than 50% women. Education success, as well as policy, participates causally in the feminization of medicine.

The reversal of the male to female medical student ratio has significant human resource policy implications. Family practitioners in Canada are still predominantly male, but this ratio is gradually reversing as the practising population ages and becomes more dominated by women (13.8% in 1978, up to 39.6% in 2009; Sarma et al., 2011). Women physicians work fewer hours, which declines further with childbearing. Younger cohorts of physicians, both male and female, as well as aging physicians of both genders, also choose to work fewer hours, seeking work-life balance. Men and women express different choices when it comes to specialty training and this variance is accentuated by the gender balance of their cohort. In a male-dominated population, female preference for the study of obstetrics and gynecology, paediatrics or family practice is magnified. In a female-dominated population (present medical school cohorts), male preference for surgery is magnified (Alers et al., 2014). In other words, gender imbalance begets greater gender imbalance and may affect delivery of specialty health care in the future. Gender balance of physician role models at higher levels is desirable, but with the pendulum of male to female student ratios in medical school swinging past the midpoint, policies encouraging or even guaranteeing gender balance in our medical schools are essential. Some have postulated that allowing a predominance of women in any one field risks creating a "pink ghetto," where that field becomes devalued, with prestige and pay following suit (Phillips, 2013).

The curriculum at Canadian medical schools has been expanded to include consideration of gender and policy issues. The AFMC has struck a resource group on equity, diversity, and gender (AFMC, 2010). This group fosters inclusiveness at the medical school level and reaches out to policymakers at the hospital and government levels. Most of the faculties of medicine in Canada have their own equity, diversity, and gender committees that influence curriculum, make policy recommendations, and examine incidences where gender equity may be threatened. In addition to addressing the climate of medical education, these groups address the working environment to assure equity in advancement and promotion, encourage opportunities for flexible work, shared jobs, and smooth flow along the off ramps and on ramps of a nonlinear career path.

While this suggests progress in identifying and policymaking to eliminate subtle or not so subtle gender bias, the effectiveness of these programs remains unclear. One study at Stanford showed that a gender sensitivity curriculum did not produce a significant decrease in gender insensitivity, but did seem to promote an inclusive workplace and a sense of well-being among women in academic medicine (Turner et al., 2012).

US Supreme Court Justice Ruth Bader Ginsburg is quoted as saying, "Now discrimination is more subtle. It's more unconscious. I think unconscious bias is one of the hardest things to get at" (Weisberg, 2014) in talking about the current obstacles facing the women's rights movement.

The academic practitioner is subject to hospital policies as well as those of the associated academic institution (university). Women leave academic medicine at much higher rates than men (Association of American Medical Colleges [AAMC], 2013). According to Gunn et al. (2014) this happens for a number of reasons, including career flexibility and incompatibility of goals for work-life balance. Hospitals lack policies that support work-life balance, and even where policies exist, senior management has little familiarity with them (Gropper et al., 2010). Levine et al. (2011) interviewed 20 women who had left academic medicine and found their reasons to be (1) lack of role models, (2) frustration with research, (3) work-life balance, and (4) institutional environment. Women are not represented at the senior management level in numbers commensurate with their representation at the faculty level. Women are less likely to be promoted even if adjusted for number of publications, amount of grant support and even hours worked (Sarma et al., 2011). This means their voice is not heard as loudly at the policy creation level and their concerns are not always addressed" (Schueller-Weidekamm & Kautzky-Willer, 2012). Absence of women at the right leadership tables results in the absence of policy for women and the absence of women.

The culture of academia is not eagerly accepting of the desire or necessity for work-life balance, which is not only relevant to Gen Xs (Cochran et al., 2013), Ys, and Zs but is rather a necessity for those women having and raising children. Seeking part time work is considered a lack of commitment (Meghen et al., 2013) by some rather than as a possible solution. Policies need to address the concerns of women as they endeavour to navigate the maze that is academic medicine, as well as the attitudes of all who are, or could be, affected by such policies. Policies for leaves, less than full-time work, and so on, need to be acceptable and used by men as well as women, particularly younger cohorts of men, as they share childrearing tasks in higher numbers. Academic productivity has been linked to appropriate and well-communicated leave policies (Gunn et al., 2014). Not only do leave policies make workplaces more productive, policies that limit work hours can benefit the health of both mothers and babies (Merchant et al., 2013).

Jerg-Bretzke and Limbrecht (2012) produced a list of possible suggestions that would make institutions, universities and hospital, more family friendly. These include (1) viewing family/work issues as a gender-independent problem, (2) providing more flexible child care provision – hours of operation and emergency availability, (3) approving flexible working hours, to include job sharing and part time, (4) creating job security, (5) loosening age limits, (6) increasing flexibility of parental leave arrangements, (7) creating more flexible career paths, (8) intensifying women-specific and family-friendly work programs, (9) building networks for support, (10) providing financial support, (11) changing thinking, such as men do more child care, and (12) redesigning corporate culture. Given that there is a will to advance in this way, many of these measures would require increased funding from provincial or territorial and federal levels, implying the development of appropriate policies at both of those levels. Our political and policy-making systems will need to be both understood and used to begin to achieve these goals. The will for change (to use new policies) and the mechanisms to bring it on, will also need to be understood.

A Story of Change

The issues demanding change are multiple and complex, as discussed at the Canadian House of Commons (Gartke & Dollin, 2010). Included here is a story of this evolution at one of Canada's largest tertiary care and academic hospitals, based on one author's experience, where the percentage of women in leadership positions mirrored the national average (13% despite making up 30% of the medical staff). In 2010, a forward-thinking CEO recognized this discrepancy and a female physician leadership committee was struck. It might be expected that progress on this front would be guaranteed and rapid with quick establishment of family-friendly policies, but change takes time regardless of the desire to embrace it.

One of the issues addressed by this committee was a perceived lack of consistent leave policies across departments and divisions. A decision was reached to examine this issue more closely and in 2011, surveys of all department heads (12) were undertaken. These surveys were personally completed by committee members in one-on-one sessions with each department head, which guaranteed 100% participation but made the process fairly unwieldy – almost a full year was required for information gathering and compilation. Surveys were supplied in advance of all interviews. The questionnaires were straightforward in asking about the existence of policies including those pertaining to parental leaves (maternity, paternity, and adoption), sick leaves, and part-time or job-share opportunities. Copies of the policies were requested. They were asked about women in their departments in leadership positions and initiatives that might encourage this.

The findings surrounding leave policies were surprising: very few department heads had any familiarity with these policies, were often not certain if they existed, and no one produced copies as requested. Four departments claimed to have a written maternity leave policy. Only one department reported a formal parental leave policy while three claimed to have something in draft and would grant unpaid leave on an ad hoc basis. One department allowed the "donation" or substitution of paid holidays for maternity leave for financial support. Only one department had a formal policy on adoption leave and no departments had policies on bereavement or elder/family care leave.

The division heads were then surveyed in 2012 – perhaps the lack of familiarity with the policies reflected the distance the department heads had from the frontlines. This was not so. The results were unchanged and a further year had passed.

In 2013, efforts to gather written copies of all the policies in existence were undertaken. After six months of fairly intensive effort, this goal was not reached. In summary then, there was significant variation among departments on the existence of leave policies, and the policies themselves were difficult to find – one department would not supply a copy and said it was "confidential." Only some of the existing policies were attached to a funding model. Most departments had no policies and some openly questioned the need for any.

In summer 2013, all hospital medical staff were sent surveys by email, in an attempt to gauge the level of importance they placed on having consistent leave policies across the institution. The response rate was approximately 30% (thought reasonably high given the season), and interestingly, of the 274 respondents, more than half were male (similar percentage as the cohort). This issue was clearly not just a women's issue.

Over 95% of responders rated maternity, bereavement, and sick leave as extremely or somewhat important. Over 80% indicated the same for paternity, parental, and caregiver leaves. About 75% placed sabbatical leave in the same category. The issue of funding for other leaves was less clear. Only 70% felt that leaves should be funded and this dropped to 62% when asked if they would be willing to contribute (by diverting the Alternate Funding Plan, monies normally shared out).

With these results in hand, through the fall of 2013, a "Suggested Guiding Principles" document was developed and adjusted with widespread input. These leave policies include pregnancy and parental leave, personal emergency leaves, personal medical leave, family medical leave, and sabbatical leave. These are often referred to as work-life policies. That document is included below and the institution's name has been redacted.

Suggested Guiding Principles Related to Work-Life Policies for Medical Staff at The * Hospital**

Access to Maternity, Paternity, Adoption, Sick and Caregiver Leaves reinforces the value that Canadians place on family and work-life balance. *** supports these values.

Active and associate medical staff at *** should enjoy the same access to Maternity, Paternity, Adoption, Sick & Caregiver Leaves as other Ontarians, in keeping with the principles of physician health and wellness. *** appointments should not be negatively impacted when members of the medical staff participate in these types of leave.

Each Department/Division should construct acceptable Work-Life Policies. These policies should abide by the guiding principles herein, and clearly specify for each type of leave:

Who is eligible

The process for requesting and approving leaves

What, if any, financial compensation is available

How coverage of medical responsibilities will be provided during the leave.

Policies should be equitably applied across the Department/ Division.

Transparency should surround all Departmental/Divisional Work-Life policies. These policies should be easily accessible. All *** physicians should be able to access them independently through "my ***" website or other secure location.

The culture surrounding access to Work-Life policies should be supportive. Department and Division heads should encourage their members to take advantage of these policies. Assistance should be readily available to clarify terms and apply the policies to individual situations. Attention should be paid to achieving equitable application of these policies across all Departments and Divisions.

Open dialogue on Work-Life policies should be encouraged at the Departmental and Divisional levels.

Feedback on Departmental/Divisional policies, to ensure that needs are being met, should be sought on a regular basis.

A formal policy was drafted including the concepts from this document of principles. Further expansion of these principles stated that the norms of provincial employment laws would be considered as minimums in terms of leave length. The leaves were expanded to include sabbaticals. Key to that document was the concept that department or division head had a responsibility to encourage and facilitate access to leaves and find solutions for coverage of clinical responsibilities. This policy was further examined at all levels of management and administration who were invited to input and finally formally accepted as hospital policy in September 2014 by the medical advisory committee. It was determined that this policy document would be posted on the hospital website and would thus be easily available to all.

De Ridder (2012) made a powerful call to action with a paper examining how to add more family to family-friendly policies. This called for a holistic approach to fundamental reforms of higher education structures – in other words, suggestions for the development of policies at the faculty level with excellent suggestions for the monitoring of success. There was a very complete list of what the policies should aim to achieve, none of which could be argued with. Changing the culture of an institution surrounding the existence and use of work-life policies remains the bigger battle. Policies may well exist but be unknown or unused (Gropper et al., 2010). If women are hesitant to seek out policies, if they feel that identifying their interest will be viewed as lack of commitment or that using leave policies will reflect negatively on their careers, then the policies will stand alone as an irrelevant monument. The problem is not so much a question of deciding policy direction but rather that even if we choose the most efficient route, change will still take years. There are many paths to culture change; the promulgation of appropriate policy is an important beginning and half the battle.

Conclusion: An Exploration of Systems Issues/Barriers to Advancement – It's Everyone's Issue

Gendered skills – can't we share?

The scarcity of women in medical leadership means that their opinions and insights are heard less at the policymaking level (Schueller-Weidekamm & Kautzky-Willer, 2012). Diversity at management levels leads to different ways of problem solving and decision making. The problems in need of solution are not "women only" problems. Women physicians may care for children and seniors disproportionately versus their male colleagues, but men are also parents and children. Parental leave is for both men and women, and both must be part of the discussion. Guilt over scheduling conflicts has no place in this life goal. Men are asking to share this responsibility: how should it be encouraged?

The winds that blow us are just as much a part of the climate of the profession as they are of personal circumstance, choice, and societal norms. Women in medicine have led the way in using personal strengths to their best advantage. Listening skills, nurturing skills, sewing skills, multitasking, and time management are not in fact gendered. These skills can be learned and shared, as much as child care can, where there is the will to do so. Do we truly believe that gender-balanced professions and gender-balanced leadership will make us stronger? Much has been done to date to describe the barriers faced by women that continue to prevent this goal. The work still to be done is in creating a climate of choice for men and women, while maximizing and using all our human talents. It will take intervention. We even have the tools.

REFERENCES

Association of American Medical Colleges. (2013). The AAMC 2011–2012 women in U.S. academic medicine and science benchmarking report. *GWIMS Watch* (Winter). Retrieved from https://www.aamc.org/download/328068/data/gwimswatchwinter2013.pdf

Association of Faculties of Medicine of Canada. (2010). Resource group on Equity Diversity and Gender Retrieved from https://afmc.ca/node/167

Association of Faculties of Medicine of Canada. (2014). *Canadian medical education statistics 2014*. Retrieved from https://www.afmc.ca/pdf/CMES2014-Complete-Optimized.pdf

Alers, M., van Leerdam, L., Dielissen, P., & Lagro-Janssen, A. (2014). Gendered specialities during medical education: a literature review.*Perspectives on Medical Education, 3*(3), 163–78. https://doi.org/10.1007/s40037-014-0132-1

Arora, S., & Galanos, A.N. (2011, Aug). The tipping point: academic careers of women in medicine today. *Academic Medicine: Journal of the Association of American Medical Colleges, 86*(8), 921–2, author reply 922. https://doi.org/10.1097/ACM.0b013e3182223054 Medline:21795896

Austin, L. (2001). *What's holding you back? Eight critical choices for women's success*. New York: Basic Books.

Bickel, J. (2001, Apr). Gender equity in undergraduate medical education: A status report. *Journal of Women's Health & Gender-Based Medicine, 10*(3), 261–70. https://doi.org/10.1089/152460901300140013 Medline:11389786

Buddeberg-Fischer, B., Stamm, M., Buddeberg, C., Bauer, G., Hämmig, O., Knecht, M., & Klaghofer, R (2010, 02 18). The impact of gender and parenthood on physicians' careers – Professional and personal situation seven years after graduation. *BMC Health Services Research, 10*(1), 40. https://doi.org/10.1186/1472-6963-10-40 Medline:20167075

Canadian Institute for Health Information. (2014). *Physicians in Canada: Summary report*. Ottawa: Author.

Cochran, A., Freischlag, J.A., & Numann, P. (2013, Apr). Women, surgery, and leadership: where we have been, where we are, where we are going. *JAMA Surgery, 148*(4), 312–13. https://doi.org/10.1001/jamasurg.2013.1706 Medline:23716118

Dageforde, L.A., Kibbe, M., & Jackson, G.P. (2013, Jan). Recruiting women to vascular surgery and other surgical specialties. *Journal of Vascular Surgery, 57*(1), 262–7. https://doi.org/10.1016/j.jvs.2012.07.029 Medline:23141685

De Ridder, D. (2012). How to add more "family" to the work-life-balance? Family friendliness in medical under- and postgraduate studies and the workplace. *GMS Z Med Ausbild, 29*(2), Doc22. Medline:22558028

Dollin, J. (2002, Jan). The feminization of family medicine: How is the health-care system influenced. *The Canadian Journal of Continuing Medical Education*, 138–45. Retrieved from http://www.stacommunications.com/journals/cme/2002/01-january/cmejan02feminization.pdf

Dollin, J. (Ed.). (2016). *The top ten skills I need to save the world*. Ottawa: Federation of Medical Women of Canada.

Duxbury, L., & Higgins, C. (2003). Work–life conflict in Canada in the new millennium. A status report Retrieved from http://publications.gc.ca/site/archivee-archived.html?url=http://publications.gc.ca/collections/Collection/H72-21-186-2003E.pdf

Dyrbye, L.N., Freischlag, J., Kaups, K.L., Oreskovich, M.R., Satele, D.V., Hanks, J.B., …, & Shanafelt, T.D. (2012, Oct). Work-home conflicts have a substantial impact on career decisions that affect the adequacy of the surgical workforce. *Archives of Surgery (Chicago, Ill.: 1960)*, *147*(10), 933–9. Medline:23117833

Eagly, A.H., Johannesen-Schmidt, M.C., & van Engen, M.L. (2003, Jul). Transformational, transactional, and laissez-faire leadership styles: A meta-analysis comparing women and men. *Psychological Bulletin*, *129*(4), 569–91. https://doi.org/10.1037/0033-2909.129.4.569 Medline:12848221

Estryn-Behar, M., Fry, C., Guetarni, K., Aune, I., Machet, G., Doppia, M.A., …, & Prudhomme, C. (2011). Work week duration, work-family balance and difficulties encountered by female and male physicians: Results from the French SESMAT study. *Work (Reading, Mass.)*, *40*(Suppl 1), S83–S100. Medline:22112665

Gartke, K., & Dollin, J. (2014). *FMWC report to the house of commons standing committee on the status of women (women in non-traditional careers)*. Retrieved from https://fmwc.ca/docs/FMWC_Report_to_the_House_of_Commons_Standing_Committee_on_the_Status_of_Women__final.pdf

Goldacre, M.J., Goldacre, R., & Lambert, T.W. (2012, Apr). Doctors who considered but did not pursue specific clinical specialties as careers: Questionnaire surveys. *Journal of the Royal Society of Medicine*, *105*(4), 166–76. https://doi.org/10.1258/jrsm.2012.110173 Medline:22532656

Gunn, C.M., Freund, K.M., Kaplan, S.A., Raj, A., & Carr, P.L. (2014, Mar-Apr). Knowledge and perceptions of family leave policies among female faculty in academic medicine. *Women's Health Issues: Official Publication of the Jacobs Institute of Women's Health*, *24*(2), e205–e210. https://doi.org/10.1016/j.whi.2013.12.008 Medline:24533979

Gropper, A., Gartke, K., & MacLaren, M. (2010, Sep). Work-life policies for Canadian medical faculty. *Journal of Women's Health (2002)*, *19*(9), 1683–703. https://doi.org/10.1089/jwh.2009.1809 Medline:20731613

Hamel, M.-B., Ingelfinger, J.R., Phimister, E., & Solomon, C.G. (2006, Jul 20). Women in academic medicine – progress and challenges. *The New England Journal of Medicine, 355*(3), 310–12. https://doi.org/10.1056/NEJMe068143 Medline:16855274

Hamilton, A.R., Tyson, M.D., Braga, J.A., & Lerner, L.B. (2012, Jun 6). Childbearing and pregnancy characteristics of female orthopaedic surgeons. *The Journal of Bone and Joint Surgery. American Volume, 94*(11), e77, 1-9. https://doi.org/10.2106/JBJS.K.00707 Medline:22637217

Heim, P. (2001). *In the company of women: Turning workplace conflict into powerful alliances*. New York: Tarcher/Putnam.

Hill, E.J.R., & Giles, J.A. (2014). *Career decisions and gender: the illusion of choice?Perspectives on Medical Education, 3*(3), 151–4. https://doi.org/10.1007/s40037-014-0128-x

Jerg-Bretzke, L., & Limbrecht, K. (2012). Where have they gone? A discussion on the balancing act of female doctors between work and family. *GMS Zeitschrift für medizinische Ausbildung, 29*(2), Doc19. Medline:22558025

Jolly, S., Griffith, K.A., DeCastro, R., Stewart, A., Ubel, P., & Jagsi, R. (2014, Mar 4). Gender differences in time spent on parenting and domestic responsibilities by high-achieving young physician-researchers. *Annals of Internal Medicine, 160*(5), 344–53. https://doi.org/10.7326/M13-0974 Medline:24737273

Knoeff, R., & Zwijnenberg, R. (Eds.). (2015). *The fate of anatomical collections (History of medicine in context)*. Farnham, England: Ashgate.

Kiolbassa, K., Miksch, A., Hermann, K., Loh, A., Szecsenyi, J., Joos, S., & Goetz, K. (2011, 05 9). Becoming a general practitioner – which factors have most impact on career choice of medical students? *BMC Family Practice, 12*(1), 25. https://doi.org/10.1186/1471-2296-12-25 Medline:21549017

Kuehn, B.M. (2012, May 9). More women choose careers in surgery: bias, work-life issues remain challenges. *JAMA, 307*(18), 1899–901. https://doi.org/10.1001/jama.2012.3725 Medline:22570448

Levine, R.B., Lin, F., Kern, D.E., Wright, S.M., & Carrese, J. (2011, Jun). Stories from early-career women physicians who have left academic medicine: A qualitative study at a single institution. *Academic Medicine, 86*(6), 752–8. https://doi.org/10.1097/ACM.0b013e318217e83b Medline:21512363

Meghen, K., Sweeney, C., Linehan, C., O'Flynn, S., & Boylan, G. (2013, Feb). Women in hospital medicine: Facts, figures and personal experiences. *Irish Medical Journal, 106*(2), 39–42. Medline:23472382

Merchant, S.J., Hameed, S.M., & Melck, A.L. (2013, Oct). Pregnancy among residents enrolled in general surgery: A nationwide survey of attitudes and experiences. *American Journal of Surgery, 206*(4), 605–10. https://doi.org/10.1016/j.amjsurg.2012.04.005 Medline:23200987

Miura, L.N., & Boxer, R.S. (2013, Jul-Aug). Women in medicine and the ticking clock. *Annals of Family Medicine, 11*(4), 381–2. https://doi.org/10.1370/afm.1515 Medline:23835825

Moss-Racusina, C., Dovidiob, J.F., Brescollc, V.L., Grahama, M.J., & Handelsmana, J. (2012). *Department of Molecular, Cellular and Developmental Biology, Department of Psychology, School of Management, and Department of Psychiatry, Science faculty's subtle gender biases favor male students*. New Haven, CT: Yale University.

National Physician Survey. (2014a). *2014 National physician survey (NPS): national demographics*. Retrieved from http://nationalphysiciansurvey.ca/wp-content/uploads/2014/10/NPS-2014-National-Demographics-EN.pdf

National Physician Survey. (2014b). *2014 National results by sex and age group – Results by topic*. Retrieved from http://nationalphysiciansurvey.ca/result/national-results-topic/

Phillips, S.P. (2013, 12 19). The growing number of female physicians: meanings, values, and outcomes. *Israel Journal of Health Policy Research, 2*(1), 47. https://doi.org/10.1186/2045-4015-2-47 Medline:24351119

Psychology Foundation of Canada. (n.d.). *Managing to manage across generations at work*. Retrieved from https://psychologyfoundation.org/Public/Resources/Workplace_Download_Resources/Public/Resources/Workplace_Download_Booklets/Workplace_Download_Resources.aspx?hkey=eed0827e-72a7-4207-a8ec-b43bef048dee

Sandler, B.R., Silverberg, L.A., & Hall, R.M. (1996). *The chilly classroom climate: A guide to improve the education of women*. Washington, DC: National Association for Women in Education.

Sarma, S., Thind, A., & Chu, M.K. (2011, Jun). Do new cohorts of family physicians work less compared to their older predecessors? The evidence from Canada. *Social Science & Medicine (1982), 72*(12), 2049–58. https://doi.org/10.1016/j.socscimed.2011.03.047 Medline:21605930

Seiden, A.M. (1989, Mar). Psychological issues affecting women throughout the life cycle. *The Psychiatric Clinics of North America, 12*(1), 1–24. Medline:2652102

Settles, I.H., Cortina, L.M., Malley, J., & Stewart, A.J. (2006). The climate for women in academic science: The good, the bad, and the changeable. *Psychology of Women Quarterly, 30*(1), 47–58. https://doi.org/10.1111/j.1471-6402.2006.00261.x

Schueller-Weidekamm, C., & Kautzky-Willer, A. (2012, Aug). Challenges of work-life balance for women physicians/mothers working in leadership positions. *Gender Medicine, 9*(4), 244–50. https://doi.org/10.1016/j.genm.2012.04.002 Medline:22626768

Shrier, D.K., & Shrier, L.A. (2009). Psychosocial aspects of women's lives: work and family/personal life and life cycle issues.*Obstetrics and Gynecology Clinics of North America, 36*(4), 753–69. https://doi.org/10.1016/j.ogc.2009.10.009

Wing Sue, D. (2010). *Microaggressions in everyday life: Race, gender, sexual orientation*. New York: Wiley.

Turner, P.L., Lumpkins, K., Gabre, J., Lin, M.J., Liu, X., & Terrin, M. (2012, May). Pregnancy among women surgeons: trends over time. *Archives of Surgery (Chicago, Ill.: 1960), 147*(5), 474–9. Medline:22351877

Valarian, V. (1998). *Why so slow: The advancement of women*. Cambridge, MA: MIT Press.

Weisberg, J. (2014, Sep 23). Supreme Court Justice Ruth Bader Ginsburg: I'm not going anywhere. *ELLE Magazine*, Retrieved from https://www.elle.com/culture/career-politics/interviews/a14788/supreme-court-justice-ruth-bader-ginsburg/

Westring, A.F., Speck, R.M., Sammel, M.D., Scott, P., Tuton, L.W., Grisso, J.A., & Abbuhl, S. (2012, Nov). A culture conducive to women's academic success: Development of a measure. *Academic Medicine, 87*(11), 1622–31. https://doi.org/10.1097/ACM.0b013e31826dbfd1 Medline:23018337

Zhuge, Y., Kaufman, J., Simeone, D.M., Chen, H., & Velazquez, O.C. (2011, Apr). Is *there still a glass ceiling for women in academic surgery? Annals of Surgery, 253*(4), 637–43. https://doi.org/10.1097/SLA.0b013e3182111120 Medline:21475000

8 Quality of Life/Life-Work Balance

SHELLEY ROSS

When I was asked to write a chapter on quality of life and worklife-homelife balance, it gave me an opportunity to reflect on my career – a career that was much more serendipitous than strategic. I am very fortunate to have had a delightful career with great personal and professional satisfaction and a very satisfactory worklife-homelife balance. If I had it all to do again, I would do so in a heartbeat.

The story goes that I knew I was going to be a doctor when I was a toddler. My uncle gave me a doctor's kit and my life's work was decided. I really had no idea what being a doctor meant as I did not come from a medical family. However, I was good in school and particularly liked the sciences and that sounded like the route for me. I never wavered in that decision but recall a time in high school when a teacher was asking the class what they planned to do. When I said medicine, she replied that nursing was a good job for a woman.

I did two years of pre-med at the University of Calgary and then had the opportunity to register in either of the two universities to which I had applied. It was Calgary's first year to run a medical school and they were using the three-year, 11-months-a-year model, so I decided to go to the University of Alberta. My reasoning was twofold: I wanted to go somewhere where they had done it before and I needed to work during the summer. Not to date myself but I was able to work as a telegraph operator and make enough money to pay my expenses for the next school year. It did help that tuition was $650 per year.

I was one of 20 females in a class of 120. The number of women admitted that year was due to Dr Odette Hagen, who took much criticism for letting so many women be admitted when the spots could have been given to men who would actually work.

The females of the class were educated like the boys, but we knew we never really were one of the boys. Great lifetime relationships were developed during our medical school years. One group in particular that felt a bond was our cadaver dissecting group. Whenever we meet at a school reunion we always talk about the good times had over our cadaver.

Being on call one in two for the third and fourth clerkship years was commonplace. I recall a psychiatrist at Edmonton General who was my preceptor, telling me that it was too bad that I was on one in two as I was missing half the good cases. Some of the cases I saw in that rotation still stay in my mind. I recall seeing a woman with catatonic schizophrenia have a reawakening following a medication injection. I also had the opportunity to visit the forensic psychiatric unit of the Alberta Hospital to use McNaughton's rule to see if the patient in question was fit to stand trial.

I recall my rotation in obstetrics. With my height being a bit under five feet, the powers that be paired me with the classmate who was six feet seven inches. The standing joke when we appeared together was here comes the short and the long of the situation. To show how things change, when I did my student obstetrics rotation, for delivery the woman's hands and feet were constrained and everyone got an episiotomy. Assessment of cervical dilatation had just been changed from a rectal exam to a vaginal exam.

I couldn't decide as time went on whether I wanted to be an obstetrician, an ophthalmologist, or a general practitioner. The decision was made when the Department of Family Practice held a wine and cheese event in fourth year and I was wooed into family medicine.

I met my husband while I was in medical school, and we married in the fall before graduation in the spring. He was working on the west coast and I hoped to find a residency there to join him. With the version of the Canadian Resident Matching System (CaRMS) that took place back then, I did not get a spot in BC on the first round. Luckily, someone decided not to take a place at the UBC Family Practice program, and I was able to spend two wonderful years connected to the relatively young UBC Family Medicine program.

As I was finishing my residency, my mother noticed an ad in the Burnaby paper looking for a doctor to work at a local full-service family practice clinic. I answered that ad and worked at that clinic for 15 years before moving my office up to the Metro town area in Burnaby, where I stayed until closing the office in 2012. I was the best example of an overachiever. I would start my day at 7 with hospital rounds, work 9 to 5:30 Monday to Friday seeing patients in the office, do paperwork half the evening, and fit in a delivery or two into the mix. The reason for closing my office was that I was becoming president of the Doctors of BC and realized I could not do justice to two masters. I did not want to be underperforming at both jobs, always finding myself in the wrong place. Since then, I have done locums in both full-service offices and maternity clinics, including intrapartum care. The interaction with patients is still a highlight of my day.

After we were married for about six years, my husband and I looked up one day and realized that we did not have any children. That problem was rectified with the birth of our first son in 1981 and our second son in 1986. My mother looked after our first son while we were working. I can remember several times when my husband was working out of town and I would get a call from the case room to come for a delivery. I would lift our son out of bed, drop him in bed between my parents who lived on the way to the hospital, and then continue onto the hospital for the delivery. We then went through a few years of trials and tribulations with nannies, so when our second son was born, my husband decided to become a house husband. He feels those were the most rewarding years of his life. When we decided to open a new office near Metrotown in Burnaby, he organized the planning and contracting of the office and then became the office manager for the medical group of six physicians until we closed it. This made him available for driving the kids back and forth to school and other activities when I had such an unreliable schedule because of the large proportion of obstetrics in my practice.

How Did I Get Involved in Organized Medicine?

When I was a second year family practice resident, the only other female in the residency program told me one day that she needed my help serving coffee, as the BC Branch of an organization known as the Federation of Medical Women of Canada (FMWC) was holding a public talk on infant nutrition featuring Dr Hedy Fry. That was my introduction to the Federation, and after serving coffee, I moved on to become president of the BC Branch, president of the national federation, president of the Medical Women's International Association (MWIA), and now secretary general of the MWIA. Dr Fry has been an MP for Vancouver Centre for many years, and whenever I see her, I tell her she was responsible for my political involvement in organized medicine.

The year that I was national president, the federation hosted the international congress of MWIA in Vancouver, and I was appointed to the Young Forum, which consisted of members under the age of 40, so you can see that age is all a matter of perspective. From Young Forum representative, I became vice president for North America and later president of MWIA.

Similarly, my involvement with the Doctors of BC (formerly the BCMA or British Columbia Medical Association) was unplanned. Unexpectedly, Dr Marshall Dahl, the representative to the board for Burnaby, asked me if I would be vice-delegate. I told him that I was much too busy, but he reassured me that I would only have to attend if he could not make a meeting and he *never* missed the meetings. After I said okay, he then decided he would run for an officer position on his way to becoming president, which made me the delegate for Burnaby. The couple of meetings a year that he referred to were actually six two-day marathons and then requests to serve on various committees.

Along the way, I was encouraged to be the chair of the board of the Doctors of BC and later the chair of the Council on Health Economics and Policy (CHEP). I was then encouraged to run for the officer positions and was uncontested the year I ran for president. When I finished as president, the chair of the General Practice Services Committee (GPSC) twisted my arm to accept the nomination for this position. Again the story went that it would only take about five days a month. In actual fact, there is never a day that I am not doing an email, a telephone call, or a meeting related to GPSC. That job then evolved into the co-chairship of the Practice Support program and its integration working group and a position on the Shared Care committee and the Joint Clinical Co-chairs committee.

At one point, at my local hospital, I was both president of the medical staff and chief of staff when the positions were combined. During that time the medical director resigned, so I did that off the side of my desk for the better part of a year. I was president of staff of the long-term-care facility in the neighbourhood. I was president of the Burnaby Medical Association, which according to many members unfortunately had become less raucous once they let the women physicians attend. When I arrived at Burnaby Hospital, there were two other women physicians on staff, both older and their involvement limited to doing rounds on their patients. So the old male guard had no idea what was going to happen when Shelley arrived and either did I.

During my time as chair of CHEP at the Doctors of BC, that position included membership in the Canadian Medical Association Council on Health Policy and Economics. Later I was appointed to CMA's Health Transformation committee. As I finished my term as president of the Doctors of BC, I was elected to be a board member of the Canadian Medical Association. Once on the board, I was elected chair of the Governance committee, which then put me on the Appointments and Review committee.

There is a rotation among the provinces and territories to provide the candidate for president-elect of the Canadian Medical Association, and 2015 was the year for BC. I threw my hat into the ring. All my work with the various committees has given me a finger on the pulse of what is happening in the world of both specialists and general practitioners. I am politically connected from my work on the collaborative committees that consist of members from both the Ministry of Health and the Doctors of BC. The job of CMA president is to speak on behalf of the organization that represents 80,000 physicians in Canada. I would have been proud to serve the 80,000 physicians in Canada, but alas it was not the time for a woman to be the president.

Choice of Specialty

Reflecting back, I realize that family medicine was the best type of practice for me. It offered the opportunity for the practice to change over time. When I first started, I saw young women and children. That suited me just fine as I was interested in women's health and particularly obstetrics and gynecology and worked my way up to doing the better part of 300 deliveries a year. As I got older, so did my patients so there was a necessity to do more internal medicine and geriatrics. I always kept a special interest in obstetrics and had a referral practice in family practice obstetrics. This had the advantage of giving me a full-service family practice with all ages but kept a young component to the practice, which many older physicians do not have. I particularly enjoyed the longitudinal aspect to the care and would have up to four generations of a family in the practice. When I was saying goodbye to my patients, it was amazing how many had been with me since birth and had never known another physician. When I became president of the Doctors of BC, I closed my practice and I now do locums in full-service family practice offices and still provide prenatal, intrapartum, and postpartum obstetric care through a variety of maternity clinics.

Quality of Life and the Doctors of BC

Much of the work I am doing at the Doctors of BC is aimed at improving the quality of life for physicians while allowing them to provide the best care for their patients. This work is done through a number of committees.

The GPSC started as a one-year project and has evolved to a collaborative committee with the Ministry of Health with a budget over $200 million yearly. It takes money negotiated through the Physician Master Agreement and puts it into areas identified as being worthy of change and quality improvement. I have co-chaired this committee with a number of Ministry of Health co-chairs.

Back in the early 2000s, there was a growing frustration among family physicians who felt that the time required to look after increasingly complex patients was not adequately compensated. Incentive fees were introduced for chronic disease management and complex care. At a time of demoralization in general practice, these incentive fees saved general practice.

GPSC has now created incentives to stop the hemorrhage of physicians that are relinquishing their acute hospital privileges and rolled out a strategy to incent excellent residential care for our frail elderly.

To encourage change in practice, GPs are allowed to bill for telephone visits up to 1500 per year. This is to discourage bringing patients into the office for follow-up advice that can safely be handled over the phone, which then frees up appointment spots for others, improving access.

Maternity care is such a rewarding part of general practice that incentive fees have been put towards ensuring its sustainability. There is concern that so few general practitioners want to incorporate obstetrics into their practice. The Maternity Care for BC incentive has been revamped to allow new GPs the opportunity to build their confidence and provide them with a mentor for a year following the program. The program is not limited to new physicians but allows a physician at any stage of his or her career to brush up their skills.

The biggest success of GPSC has been the development of the Divisions of Family Practice. As physicians left the hospital setting, there was nowhere in the community to share ideas and support one another or to interact with the health authorities. The Divisions took on a huge initiative, known as AGPforMe, which is also known as the Attachment Initiative. The goal was threefold: allowing those who want a GP to find one, strengthening the relationship for those who have a GP but do not fully access their care through that GP, and providing care for vulnerable patients. Although not every BC resident got a family doctor, many did and many were prevented from being orphaned when their physician retired by attaching them elsewhere. Much of what was learned is being used as we develop the Patient Medical Home and Primary Care Network.

I have also been fortunate to sit on the Shared Care committee, another collaborative committee between the Doctors of BC and the Ministry of Health. This committee has concentrated on projects to help general practitioners and specialists work better together.

My favourite project originating from this committee is tele-dermatology. In BC, it can be months before a patient can see a dermatologist. With this program, you take a picture of the skin lesion with your smart phone and send it through a secure site to dermatologists who come back with a diagnosis and treatment plan within 48 hours.

Another success story is RACE which stands for Rapid Access to Consultative Expertise. There is a single phone number that gives the general practitioner access to advice from a specialist from a vast number of specialties, often within an hour.

The biggest project for Shared Care is the Child and Youth Mental Health and Substance Abuse Collaborative. Too often we hear of children and youth with mental health issues who cannot access the care they require. This collaborative has brought together every player in child and youth mental health and builds trust among partners as they change the system for the betterment of our young patients. The Doctors of BC (2014) wrote a paper on mental health, entitled *Reaching Out: Supporting Youth Mental Health in British Columbia,* and have developed a website entitled OpenMindBC.ca to provide access to mental health tools and resources. The Practice Support program has developed training modules on both child and youth and on adult mental health to train general practitioners on best practice. Although the collaboration has ended, three legacy tracks continue, namely, ACES (adverse childhood experiences), inter-ministry collaboration with physicians, and support for local action teams, which bring all stakeholders together to improve the local situation.

I co-chaired the Practice Support program mentioned above. In addition to clinical training modules, the program is providing practice coaching. With the General Practice Services Committee engaged in leading the Patient Medical Home work and substantially influencing the Primary Care Network work, the PSP is essential in supporting physicians with coaching and helping them with a variety of activities that allow them to understand their patient panel, start to work in teams, form physician networks and work with the Primary Care Network.

Quality of Life and Generational Change

How often have you heard doctors from the baby boomer generation (born 1946 to 1964) complain about the new generation – it will take three of the new grads to do the work I do, they are not interested in anything but lifestyle, what happened to dedication and the good old days? These comments offer a bit of catharsis but are not helpful for moving forward. Those planning for the future have to realize that ideas have changed.

I had the opportunity to attend a workshop held for the board of the Canadian Medical Association on Generations X and Y. It is apparent that the baby boomers have had it their way for a long time. The fact is that 53% of the population now is either Generation X (1965–1981) or Generation Y (1982–2005), and their values are going to replace the values of those baby boomers currently in the leadership positions (Sladek, 2014).

These redefined values have required redefining the culture of organizations. The approach to work has changed in that what defines success now is the degree of satisfaction that work brings. Organizations need to offer what others cannot and save time which is the most precious commodity. For those looking at the future of health care delivery, Generations X and Y are going to make up the majority of the workforce, so we need to realize that new values are redefining how we work.

This is not to say that those entering medicine are any less dedicated but they are much smarter in protecting their time than the baby boomers were. What makes people go into medicine is no different from one generation to another.

Medicine is a calling, not a means to a good-paying job. Wherever I go, I run into patients. It is delightful to make contact and to know that you have made such an impact on people's lives that they recognize you after many years. I once had a new couple come to the office for a first prenatal visit. When I asked how they had found me, the husband stated that I had delivered him 30 years ago and now with his wife was pregnant, he remembered my name.

Although we are much more aware of the balance between work and home, we must make sure that we don't hear the comment I heard a few years ago – "I don't want to be thought of as a doctor – I am a person whose job is a doctor!" Once you become a doctor, you are always a doctor. Being a physician is a privilege. What other job gives you so many positives: influence, self-regulation, the ability to positively influence peoples' lives, satisfaction in the job, variety and generally having the respect of the public. The doctor patient relationship is so important. There is an art to making patients feel that they are the most important thing in your day when you are looking after them.

I have been asking various physicians how they manage worklife-homelife balance. For some, there is no management. They feel that they are on a treadmill, barely able to keep up with the day-to-day activities with no time to plan for balance. Others say that they periodically take a step back and see if what they are doing relates to what they want from life and if does not, they make changes. One particularly philosophical physician told me that she looks at balance like the *Canada Food Guide*. On that guide are categories like work, family, exercise, time to write, time for leisure, to give a few examples. She needs to make sure that she selects a certain number of activities from each category each day, and if she finds she is deficient in a category she makes sure she increases her selections from that category. No matter how they manage balance, whether well or not, it is top of mind for many physicians.

Women in Medicine

Going beyond the Generation X and Y discussion is the discussion around the number of women in medicine. Rather than realizing that it is a generation – involving both men and women – that expect different things than the baby boomers, there is a great deal of finger pointing at women in medicine being the root of all evil. The *pink collar profession* and the *feminization of medicine* are words that have negative connotations.

Having said that however, the educational process for medicine is long and those graduating are in their prime reproductive years. Too often we see problems of infertility because female physicians have left their plans for pregnancy behind as they advance through their years of training. The biological responsibility for pregnancy rests with the woman; however, there is the ability for both partners to share in the responsibilities of childrearing. Medical associations have recognized this dual responsibility by changing maternity benefits to parental benefits. The realization that physicians are going to become pregnant and have children and then have responsibilities in raising those children must be factored into the development of any staffing plan. With the arrival of children comes competing demands for physicians' time.

Lynda Buske, when she was with the Canadian Collaborative Centre for Physician Resources of the Canadian Medical Association, looked at the analysis of workload trends among Canadian physicians. The gap in hours worked between male and female physicians is narrowing. Female physicians who are also mothers clearly demonstrate that they have a second shift of work in childcare compared to their male counterparts. For physicians with no children, there is only a minor difference in workload between males and females. Time spent providing direct patient care is continuing to decline for both genders but the time required to complete paperwork is increasing (Buske, 2011).

Lynda Buske goes on to report on the analysis of physician professional satisfaction within the National Physician Survey. The same cohorts were followed from year to year. In these cohorts, there was a correlation between both fewer hours worked and a shift away from fee for service and increased satisfaction. Longer working hours cutting into free time led to dissatisfaction (Buske, 2013).

According to Canadian Institute for Health Information (2013), between 2009 and 2013, the number of female physicians increased by 22.5%, while the number of male physicians increased by 9.2%.

As of 2014, women made up 42.2% of general practitioners in the country but only 33.9% of specialists. There are some specialties like pediatrics (54.7%) in which women are in the majority. Many of the surgical specialties have shown an increased number of women, but urology and orthopedic surgery are still well under 10% (Canadian Medical Association, 2015). Of the 77,479 active physicians in Canada in 2014, 47,941 were women and 29,538 were men (Canadian Medical Association, 2015). The trend shows that women are becoming a larger number of the new medical graduates. In 1968, 10% of the MD degrees granted in Canada were granted to women. In 1974, the year I graduated, it had jumped to 20%. In 2012, this number had changed to 58.3% (Canadian Medical Association, 2014).

The Federation of Medical Women of Canada and the Medical Women's International Association

Both FMWC and MWIA date back to a time when women were by far the minority of the physician workforce. MWIA was started in 1919 by

Dr Esther Pohl Lovejoy of the United States, along with international colleagues. FMWC was founded in 1924 by Dr Maude Abbott, a friend and colleague of Sir William Osler, and world renowned for her work on congenital heart disease.

The main concern in the early stages of these organizations was the difficulty women had in being able to attend medical school. The organizations advocated for the right of women to attend medical school and to practise medicine. With the number of women graduating from medicine in Canada in 2014 at 58.3%, I think these organizations can be congratulated on achieving their goals.

You will recall my earlier comment that although we were trained like the boys, we were never really one of the boys. The same holds true today when it comes to medical leadership positions for women. If the majority of new graduates are women, where are the women in leadership positions? The higher up the hierarchy you go; the fewer women you find. Canada saw its first two female deans of medical schools only a few years ago, Dr Noni MacDonald for Dalhousie and Dr Carole Herbert for Western. So often women in medicine feel there is no gender discrimination. In the day-to-day practice of medicine, this is often true, but once you start to show interest in a leadership position, things change. Women do not always support other women and sometimes can be their biggest opponents. Women often forget to bring other women up the leadership ladder with them as they advance.

With membership from over 70 countries, MWIA provides a means of meeting women physicians from different parts of the world. Such meetings show that no matter how much we may be culturally different, we are all the same with our challenges as women in medicine. It is a great organization for networking with women physicians from around the world. Having a personal connection with a physician changes the interaction with that physician when required on a business level.

In addition to advocating for women in medicine, another role of the FMWC and MWIA is advocating for women's health. Leaving the day-to-day work of medicine in Canada and seeing the challenges of medicine elsewhere are life changing.

I recall touring the public maternity hospital in Nairobi back in the early 1990s. There were so many women in labour that all the skilled attendants could manage was to run to deliver one woman after another as the head was crowning. Monitoring of labour and the use of partograms were unheard of luxuries. I recall a row of women sitting on a bench and when I enquired as to what they were doing, the answer was that they were waiting for suturing of their episiotomies. I had the opportunity to tour the same hospital 15 years later and the only change was that now one-third of the patients were HIV positive. It was not uncommon to see two labouring women sharing one bed and I recall one woman shouting at her bedmate, demanding that she move over so that her blood did not get on her.

MWIA has taken quite an interest in the eradication of female genital mutilation. When there were a number of Somali refugees arriving in greater Vancouver, many of them settled in Burnaby. I was able to put my international knowledge to practical use when de-infibulation was required for delivery.

The medical women are well known for their work on gender and health. This is defined as more than just the biological differences between women and men. The two other important aspects to gender and health are the societal and cultural norms (what society feels is normal behaviour for men and for women), and the power relations between men and women. In addition to a training manual on gender, MWIA has another training manual on adolescent sexuality, and one on gender based violence. All can be found on the website at https://www.mwia.net.

MWIA is in official relations with the World Health Organization, has Category II status with the Economic and Social Council of the United Nations, and is a member of the NGO branch of the UN Department of Public Information. This gives members the opportunity to have non-governmental organization input on global public policy and to see the workings of international organizations.

FMWC and MWIA offer a collective voice on issues such as female genital mutilation, gender based violence, cosmetic genital surgery, and safe childbirth. MWIA is currently partnering with Zonta to provide safe birthing kits to refugee camps for locally displaced persons in Afghanistan and for primary health centres in Nigeria. The collective voice offers more hope for advocacy for women's health than a lone voice.

Vision of the Future for Primary Care

I frequently hear from physicians what it is that gives them a sense of satisfaction with the job: a good quality of life and worklife-homelife balance. One of the biggest factors leading to less job satisfaction is the shortage of physicians, which translates into more work for those on the ground. Doctors like to work but they also want dedicated time off. The day of the solo practitioner is over. Although we hear the word *teamwork* as the answer to patient care of the future, the idea of a team is different to many people.

The first kind of team is a team of family doctors working together. I have heard the suggestion that a good size for a group of family doctors is nine. Having a group of nine allows for one night a week on call, with a couple of spares when people are unavailable. General practitioners need to keep a broad base to their practice, and if they have a special interest it should be on a background of this broad based general practice. In a group of nine, there could be a number of special interests – obstetrics, geriatrics, dermatology, respiratory, palliative care – to name a few. This would allow referral for difficult cases within the practice with less dependence on hard-to-access specialists.

The other type of team is the various allied health personnel that are needed to provide patient care. This team varies from patient to patient, making it difficult to house the team in one location. What is needed is a seamless flow back and forth from the GP's office for the various services. Community care, ambulatory care, hospital care, and care in the specialist's office should all be easily accessible to a practice without long waits.

This concept flows into the idea of the Patient Medical Home. The GPSC conducted a visioning process around the province, asking GPs how they saw the future and how they wanted to practise in that future world. What was heard was translated into the Patient Medical Home, based on the College of Family Physicians of Canada Patient Medical Home, but with a BC twist. With the patient at the centre, the PMH is wrapped around the patient and there are the service attributes like comprehensiveness, coordination, and access and the relationship attributes like teams of physicians and teams with allied health professionals, with supports like IT, research, and teaching. Attribute number 12 is the team of physicians and allied health professions that translates into BC's Primary Care Network.

Recruitment and Retention of Family Physicians

If physicians are to have good quality to life, there needs to be enough physicians to share the workload. The presentations by Divisions of Family practice in the AGPforMe program inevitably had recruitment and retention as one strategy. When I would raise my hand and ask from where they are recruiting, the answer was unclear. Further investigation shows that the biggest pool of recruits is new family practice residents. Other sources are physicians working elsewhere in the country and physicians from Ireland, the United Kingdom, the United States, and Australia, which have reciprocity with the College of Family Physicians of Canada.

Twenty to 30 years ago the group of doctors who wanted to come to Canada were the South Africans. They were well trained, had lots of rural experience as well as experience in advanced disease, and after a while had enough other South Africans for neighbours to make them feel at home. While touring BC during my time as President of the Doctors of BC, the more rural and remote the community, the more the South African influence. In one community, 95% of the doctors were South African, causing a complaint to be made that Afrikaans was being spoken in the operating room!

The group that wants to come to Canada now is the Canadians studying abroad (CSAs). CSAs are Canadian citizens who went abroad to study medicine. International medical graduates (IMGs) are defined as having received their medical training before arriving in Canada and receiving Canadian citizenship. In years gone by, CSAs trained in like-minded countries could apply for a residency back home. Because of a human rights complaint some years ago, CSAs are considered a subset of IMGs. Although trained internationally, they are Canadians with an understanding of the Canadian system and culture.

I was involved in developing a summit on recruitment and retention that will tackle the CSA problem as well as the numerous other hurdles that doctors face when trying to practice in BC. All stakeholders have been involved, and the outcome of the summit was threefold: (1) the development of practiceinbc.ca website with all the information and links necessary to navigate the system for those wanting to come to BC or for doctors or communities in BC wanting to find a permanent or locum doctor; (2) a sharing of best practices with clear outline of what the responsibility is at the local, regional, and provincial level; and (3) the creation of the GPSC Provincial Recruitment and Retention Committee, which I co-chair, that involves all organizations that touch or influence recruitment and retention in the province, to allow a proactive rather than reactive response to physician manpower needs.

Recommendations

As I reflect back over my last 40 years in the field of medicine, I would like to summarize in 10 points the things that I found were important to having worklife-homelife balance, a good quality of life, and professional satisfaction.

1. Pick Your Partners Carefully

This refers to both your life partner and your working partners. I could not have done half of what I have without such a supportive husband. I would go further to say that it takes a whole family to support one person in medicine. When women in medicine marry other professionals who are advancing up the career ladder, it is usually the woman who finds herself as the supporting person. This means that her career could be limited in scope and opportunities. This requires thoughtful discussion and decision between the partners.

The other partners are your working partners. If you are going to be involved in activities that take you away from the office or other medical duties, you need colleagues who will cover for you when you are out of the office or scheduled to be on call. Your colleagues need to believe that by increasing their workload to support you that what you are doing is for the good of all. It is great to have a reliable locum, but locums are something of a past luxury. If your colleagues are not supportive, it leads to ongoing tensions for all concerned.

2. Make Time for Your Entire Family

One of the most important jobs I have listed in my CV is that of being a wife, a mother, and now a grandmother. Family must be your first priority as they will be there for you through thick and thin. You can believe that your work as a doctor is so important that you put it before family. While family will need you and support you forever, the same is not true for patients. When working life is finished, it is like taking your hand out of water – there is no sign that you have been there.

Make sure you stay involved in the family's activities. Celebrate the important occasions. Volunteer at the school. I was the homeroom mother for the grade 3 class. I then had the advantage of knowing all the parents and kids for the rest of the school years. In the effort to make time for family activities, don't forget to make time for your partner. Do things as a couple, and remember that a relationship needs constant nurturing and should not be taken for granted.

3. Make Efficient Use of Your Time

Take stock of how you use your time, both at home and in the office. Don't be doing tasks that could be delegated to others. At home, a prime example is getting help with the housework. Having your house clean and in order is great, but no one is watching to make sure you do it yourself. You could be using that time to spend with your family doing things that are fun and memorable. Another example is how you handle your mail. I deal with the mail in one handling. When the mail arrives, I sort through it once. The junk mail is immediately is thrown away and what needs action is readied for that action. Shifting through the mail and putting it back down on the counter means that you have to keep resorting it over and over, which is a waste of time.

There is no shortage of examples of office inefficiencies but I have chosen two that I have seen repeatedly. The first example is that physicians think they are saving money by doing clerical work themselves. As a physician do what physicians need to do, and have others do work that you do not need to do. As a physician, you need to have patient interaction to diagnose and treat. If you are spending your time in doing tasks such as phoning for appointments, you are doing work that others can do. The second example is charting. By the time you finish the patient interaction, the charting should be finished. Leaving documentation until the end of the day is exhausting and inefficient because you cannot remember all that went on during the patient visit, and this makes the entry much more time-consuming, not to mention inaccurate.

You must be open to stepping back and looking at how you do things and then be willing to make changes. There is help out there (take the example of practice coaching through the Doctors of BC Practice Support program) to assist you in making the necessary changes to ensure that your office runs efficiently. One way to try new things is the PDSA (plan, do, study, act) cycle, which allows you to implement new ways of doing things and then evaluate changes before making the changes permanent.

4. Stop Saying No and Start Saying Yes

The majority of leadership positions I enjoyed came not because I went looking for them but because someone asked me to do something in organized medicine. I notice that over the last few years there has been considerable training to say no and not get involved, in the name of worklife-homelife balance. However, after a number of times saying no, you will find you aren't asked again. Not for a moment am I suggesting that you say yes to every offer that comes your way, but if there is an issue that you are passionate about and the opportunity to get involved arises, don't let it slip by.

Also, remember that if you wish to champion a cause, your voice is much louder if it is added to the collective voices of others. Originally, the FMWC and MWIA were started to advocate for women in medicine and to get women into medical school. With so many women in medicine now, the focus needs to change to make sure we train women to take on the higher leadership roles. The other role of FMWC and MWIA is to champion issues in women's health. Take the relatively recent example of the getting HPV vaccine covered in the schools – that was accomplished under the leadership of Dr Gail Beck when she was president of the federation. No other organization would take on the issue, but the federation realized it was the right thing to do and didn't give up until it happened.

5. *Stand Up, Speak Up, and Shut Up*

Once you have said yes to becoming involved, be good for your word. If you say you are going to do something, then make sure you do. There are certain skills you will need. One of these skills is being able to present your thoughts in a clear, concise, and convincing manner. Make sure you don't whine as it alienates people and is counterproductive.

Another skill is how to run a meeting efficiently. One thing that is even more important than starting on time is finishing on time. One trick to getting people to arrive on time is to start on time with the most important business first. Do not penalize the punctual. Know your rules of order but be flexible enough to let the work get done. You need to have emotional intelligence and be able to read the mood of the group.

A third skill is how to deal with the media. If you want to get your message out to the public, you need to overcome your fear of being interviewed. Make sure you develop these skills and others early on and get training if it does not come naturally.

6. *Mentor and Be Mentored*

I had two great mentors in my career. One was a male obstetrician who loved to teach general practitioners and gave me skills that made my career in family practice obstetrics so much more enjoyable. My other outstanding mentor was Dr May Cohen. May is a professor emeritus in the Department of Family Practice at McMaster and is known for her advocacy for gender equality, women's health, and sexual health. I had the great pleasure in the early 2000s of writing two training manuals with her for MWIA. One was on gender mainstreaming in health and the other on adolescent sexuality. Mentoring is not all about clinical medicine but can include practical everyday answers, such as how to manage a career and family. To take mentoring to the next level, there are physicians available that have training in career coaching.

As a physician, whether you are in an official mentoring role or not, you are a role model for other women in medicine and other allied health care professionals. When you mentor others, you gain as much as you give. Always treat people the way you would like to be treated. As the leader of the team, look after your team members, make their life better, and ensure they have the opportunity to advance and learn. Don't make it all about you.

7. Be a Lifelong Learner

What you learn in medical school is just a taste of what you need to practise medicine. Make sure that you keep current in what is changing in medicine but also expand your knowledge to fields outside of medicine. I had the opportunity recently to do a board directors course at the Rotman School of Management in Toronto. I was in a class of 40 business people – managing partners of law firms and accounting firms, vice presidents of the major banks and credit unions, those in charge of pension funds – you get the idea. There were three other doctors – one in a public health leadership role, one who was a CEO of a hospital, and one who had developed medical record storage in the cloud. I have never felt so out of place in my life. However, the course talked about such things as what board governance is versus management, audit committees, dealing with the CEO, learning what makes an effective board, – things I have found useful countless times since I finished the course. The best thing I learned about governance was NIFO – noses in and fingers out. Leave management to do the micromanagement, but as a board of governors give them direction and ensure that they deliver. The lesson I learned is don't be afraid to learn something new, surrounded by a different group of people. While speaking of education, remember to also take courses that are fun. It is good to cultivate other interests.

8. Be Passionate and Don't Be Afraid to Dig in Your High Heels

You need to believe in things, be passionate, and have a fearless heart. In the world of women's health, it is amazing how women suffer needlessly. In the comfortable world into which we were lucky to be born, we must not become complacent. Many say feminism is dated and it may be for the privileged but not for the majority of women. We need to stand up for those who cannot stand up for themselves. It starts with taking paths that are not always popular and not being afraid to stick to your convictions. Use your emotional intelligence to realize that just because you feel passionately about a topic, you still have to get people to buy in and support and follow you. You need to have social awareness to read what impact your argument is having on others. Corporations are realizing that people skills are as important in a CEO as technical and management knowledge. Make sure you have done your homework before you get to a meeting where a vote will occur. There is nothing worse than to feel the political wind blowing in the direction opposite to what you want to achieve.

As a leader you are responsible for setting the tone at the top. Keep your values high and let those who work with you realize that you expect the same from them. There must be a culture of excellence in your organizations.

Be loyal to whatever organization you belong to. You will often find that members of the Federation or MWIA stay loyal to the organization for a lifetime. These organizations offer women a safe place to learn how to be leaders, and they feel a sense of belonging.

9. Remember That You Will Never Be One of the Boys

When I went to medical school, I was one of 20 women in a class of 120. How things have changed! We were educated like our male colleagues, partied with them, did the med show together, and felt we were one of the crowd. Similarly, when you get involved in organizations, as a woman you sit in the minority around a board table and think you are on an equal footing with the guys. However, a funny thing happens when an important position comes up and both women and men are competing for the position. Men support one another and push the male candidate forward, whereas women are not so good at that. There was a past president of the American Medical Women's Association who often said that you need to identify men of good conscience. By that she meant men that believed women were just as capable as men and would advocate for them.

10. Look after Yourself and Lead by Being Seen

There is so much more to being a physician than just the practice of medicine. You need to get involved and support the people with whom you associate. You need to be calm, dependable, and in charge when the need arises. If you let yourself panic in times of stress, who is going to be in control? You are a pillar of the community and need to act accordingly. Look the part of a physician – dress properly, and conduct yourself in a becoming manner. But more than that, look after your own health. Incorporate some exercise into your day, eat properly, get enough sleep, find the worklife-homelife balance that suits you and your family, learn how to deal with stress, and in the spirit of cognitive behavioural therapy, make sure you stay positive. Take enough vacation time. Add variety to your life by getting involved in activities outside the day-to-day grind of the office. There are so many opportunities for meaningful involvement.

Physicians need to remember that to those to whom much is given, much is expected in return. I think of the years that I worked with the case room and postpartum staff. I attended Christmas parties, retirements, and baby showers, and learned how to knit and do crosswords – all with the staff. I stood up for those I worked with when the going would get tough. I made myself visible. I recall a talk by Major General Lewis MacKenzie, commander of the UN Protection Force in Sarajevo, who said that he would get out and walk among the troops every day so that they knew he was there. You need to lead by being present.

In conclusion, I doubt my career could have been any more enjoyable if I had actually had a strategic career plan instead of a career determined by serendipity. Considering worklife-homelife balance, I have come through a busy career still with the same husband of over 40 years, a happy, connected family, and an excellent quality of life. I have been fortunate to have it all. I can only wish the same for every woman in medicine!

REFERENCES

Buske, L. (2011). *Trends in physician workload based on survey data*. Ottawa: Canadian Medical Association.

Buske, L. (2013). *Analysis of physician professional satisfaction within the national physician survey cohort*. Ottawa: Canadian Collaborative Centre for Physician Resources, Canadian Medical Association.

Canadian Medical Association. (2014). *Number of MDs awarded by Canadian universities by sex, 1968–2016*. Retrieved from https://www.cma.ca/Assets/assets-library/document/en/advocacy/25-MD_awarded_by_sex.pdf

Canadian Medical Association. (2015). *Number and percent distribution of physicians by specialty and sex, Canada*. Retrieved from https://www.cma.ca/Assets/assets-library/document/en/advocacy/06SpecSex.pdf

Canadian Institute for Health Information. (2013). Physicians in Canada: Summary report. Ottawa: Author.

Doctors of BC. (2014). *Reaching out: Supporting youth mental health in British Columbia*. Retrieved from https://www.doctorsofbc.ca/policy-papers/reaching-out-supporting-youth-mental-health-british-columbia

Sladek, S. (2014). *Knowing Y*. Washington, DC: The Center for Association Leadership.

SECTION FOUR

Contemporary Perspectives on Women in Medicine

We are living in a time of constant change. Advances in medicine and the increasing influence of information technology have had a profound impact on how medicine is (and will be) practised. Internal and external pressures, most particularly the changing expectations of patients who are better informed (or misinformed, as the case may be), are modifying the physician work situation completely. While those outside the profession may hold that these are all easily incorporated into the profession, in fact they may suggest rapid changes and even dramatically different activity for the practitioner. Contemporary medical practice is held to high standards, with the public assuming that new procedures and knowledge can be quickly incorporated into the doctor's environment. In this section, we present multiple perspectives on the ways in which contemporary medicine is changing and how those changes are both influenced by and have an influence on the experiences of female physicians. In Chapter 9, Erin Fredericks presents an academic overview of how female physicians approach ethical decision making. In Chapter 10, Monica Olsen, Mamta Guatam, and Gillian Kernaghan discuss the unique challenges faced by female physicians, and how new ways to approaching individual practice and the structure of systems can be leveraged to improve experiences of both physicians and patients. Finally, in Chapter 11, Perle Feldman gives a personal account of how the practice of medicine has changed in the course of her career, how female physicians may have had an influence on how physicians interact with patients, and how patient expectations have been shaped by their experiences with the differences in practice between male and female physicians.

9 Women Physicians as Ethical Decision Makers

ERIN FREDERICKS

Introduction

While a significant number of empirical studies have examined the experiences of women working in medicine, far fewer have engaged with the ways in which the increasing number of women physicians have changed medical practice and, in particular, the ethical dimensions of this practice. As more women enter the field of medicine, scholars and practitioners have debated how women physicians will change medicine. Some have raised concerns that women will work fewer hours (College of Family Physicians of Canada [CFPC], 2010), see fewer patients, and take more time off for family issues (Biringer & Childress, 2012) and that this decrease in patient care will damage the profession. These claims have been critiqued for being sexist and some critics have demonstrated this is not the case (Herbert et al., 2008).

In contrast, some scholars and physicians have wondered if increasing gender diversity among physicians will humanize or improve medical practice (Riska, 2001) by increasing the caring, empathetic, and patient-centred care patients receive in the clinic and more broadly in decision making about what medical practice should be. Despite the fact that both claims that women will ruin or humanize medicine rely on an assumption that women physicians are innately different and naturally more nurturing than men, the latter claim is not as often deemed sexist. Whether women physicians are criticized for the nurturing they provide children at home that distracts from their practices or praised for the nurturing they provide patients in the clinic that improves patient care, a particular image of women physicians is being forwarded: women physicians are seen to be naturally caring.

Intuitively, it seems probable that women physicians make distinctive ethical decisions. A number of empirical studies have supported this intuition by concluding that women physicians are more likely to show an interest in learning about ethics and ethical principles (Roberts et al., 2004; Roberts et al., 2005), spend more time with patients (Levinson & Lurie, 2004), develop collaborative relationships with their patients, and engage patients in discussions of complex psychosocial issues (Heru, 2005). However, studies have also demonstrated that professional socialization (Beagan, 2000) and structural constraints, such as lack of representation in upper level positions, may limit women physicians and their effects on medical practice (Heru, 2005; McKinstry et al., 2006; Riska, 2001) Further, some women physicians have been shown to be less satisfied with their work, and this could, in part, be a result of the emotional labour involved in these approaches to ethical practice.

At the same time, debates about what it means to practise ethically are taking place in academia, medical schools, and clinics. This debate centres on whether ethical decisions should be based on an abstract set of principles that physicians learn to apply to diverse cases, or whether an alternative approach is required to address the increasing complexity of ethical decision making given competing demands on the physician and increasing use of technology (Hafferty & Franks, 1994). Principlism, represented in the work of Beauchamp and Childress (2001) suggests that ethical decisions must reflect the principles of beneficence, autonomy, justice, and non-maleficence. Although few have suggested these principles be disregarded altogether, alternative ethical frameworks have suggested approaches to ethics that prioritize narrative or care, or better attend to power relations, among others.

It is beyond the scope of this chapter to argue that one of these competing ethical frameworks is morally superior. As a sociologist, I am less concerned with which framework is best and more concerned with understanding the social construction of women physicians as ethical or unethical decision makers. In this chapter, I examine approaches to ethical decision making that are seen as characteristically feminine or common among women physicians, and the effects of our views of women physicians as potentially distinctive ethical decision makers.

What Does It Mean to Be a Woman?

In our society, we have ideas about what it means to be a woman. In comparison to men, women are often thought to be physically weaker, worse at math and sciences, and more irrational. These ideas have been countered because they demean women in relation to men, but they persist in many taken-for-granted ways and shape our interactions with others. We also have ideas about women that are deemed positive characteristics. We see women as more nurturing, empathetic listeners, and more apt to care for others. Outside of feminist scholarship, these ideas are countered less often because they are seen to be less insulting to women and better account for our experiences of women in our lives. However, from a sociological perspective, all taken-for-granted understandings about members of a social group have both enabling and constraining effects. In other words, believing women are more nurturing than men is not just complimentary – it also constrains women and shapes their social interactions.

At this point, it will be useful to examine where these ideas come from. In our society, it is commonly believed that many of our characteristics as individuals are rooted in our biology. That is, many behavioural characteristics are seen as innate, biological attributes. This is referred to as biological determinism, the assumption that human behaviour is based primarily in biology and thus is predetermined. Similarly, essentialism refers to the idea that there are essential differences between members of different social groups (whether or not these are based in biology). From an essentialist and biological deterministic view, women are understood to be naturally different from men.

Biological studies of sex-based differences between men and women demonstrating women to be the "weaker sex" have been used to justify the exclusion of women from politics, mathematics and sciences, and other positions of power while keeping women relegated to private spaces, such as the home. However, some research counters this biological determinism and demonstrates that women and are men not significantly different in their biology, and further counters the existence of two binary genders (Fausto-Sterling, 1992). Despite evidence that women are not naturally different from men and that our binary gender system is socially constructed and not natural, we continue to experience gender difference as very real.

Sociological and other alternative perspectives on gender describe gender differences as consequences of socialization and social experiences, not innate biological characteristics. Socialization is the process of becoming a social being or member of society. Individuals learn how to behave through interactions with others. In other words, in the case of gender, babies are born, assigned the label of "male" or "female" (in most cases), and then treated differently based on this label. Through social interactions and cultural expectations in the form of social norms, women learn and perform the gender role of "woman." This does not mean that gender is entirely social, but there is significant evidence that much of what we view as natural differences between women and men are actually socially constructed.

All individuals are socially located, meaning that their membership in particular social groups shapes their perspectives. Whether or not these individuals explicitly identify with a social group, their membership in these groups influences their experiences and views (Beagan, 2000). For groups that are oppressed, such as women, experiences of discrimination are among those that shape the world views of these individuals. Simone de Beauvoir (1972 [1949], p. 18) suggested that "social discrimination produces in women moral and intellectual effects so profound that they appear to be caused by nature." In other words, in comparison to men, women have particular social experiences that shape who they are, how they act, how they treat others, and how others treat them. Within the social group of women, individuals will also have varied experiences of oppression and world views because of their membership in other social groups.

Social constructions (like gender) are not real in a natural or biological sense, but they are real in their consequences. It may not be biologically true that women are naturally worse at math than men, but because teachers, students, and parents often believe this is true, girls tend to score lower on math exams. The effects of social constructions are produced by complex social interactions that reproduce social roles and norms.

Similarly, the idea that women are more nurturing seems correct because women learn to be more nurturing or are assumed to be more nurturing, and thus others go to them to be nurtured. For women physicians, this gendered expectation of care has led to the divergent arguments that women may be worse physicians because they are too caring to make tough decisions or too distracted by their private lives, or better physicians because they are more caring and spend more time in discussion with patients.

These debates about women as carers are not framed as disagreements about ethical practice, but in many ways they are about moral reasoning. Arguments that women physicians are too caring to make tough decisions contain a concern that women physicians may be less likely to act on the ethical principle of justice, which sometimes requires that the known patient does not benefit from a decision. Reports that women physicians are more caring and communicative in patient care may suggest that women physicians are more likely to act on the ethical principle of beneficence. When women physicians are described as having essentially different practice styles, these descriptions have distinct ethical implications.

Arguments about the characteristics of women physicians and their practice are complicated by studies of professional socialization that demonstrate that medical school may train people from diverse social categories to act in similar ways. Beagan (2000), for example, demonstrates that physicians from diverse social groups become "neutral" providers through medical training. In other words, professional medical socialization may counter some of the socially constructed differences between men and women by requiring physicians to develop an impartial perspective. However, there is no such impartial knowledge; knowledge is constructed from a particular perspective, and seemingly impartial knowledge actually reflects the perspective of dominant groups (Beagan, 2000; Haraway, 1991; Harding, 1993). Dominant conceptions of ethics, for example, have been criticized for privileging values commonly deemed masculine, such as justice and autonomy (Tong, 1993).

Ethical Decision Making

Scholars, educators, and physicians draw on different definitions of ethics, and diverse ethical frameworks. Pojman (1990) provides a definition of traditional ethics as the

> systematic endeavour to understand moral concepts and justify moral principles and theories. It undertakes to analyze such concepts as "right," "wrong," "permissible," "ought," "good," and "evil" in their moral contexts. Ethics seeks to establish principles of right behaviour that may serve as action guides for individuals or groups. It investigates which values and virtues are paramount to the worthwhile life or to society. (p. 2)

Ethical frameworks provide principles for good action and virtue, which actors must then use in practice. While there are diverse approaches to ethics, one has come to dominate health care practice. In health care, the most common ethical framework is principlism, which refers to the use of abstract principles to make moral decisions. Beauchamp and Childress's (2001) four ethical principles, autonomy, beneficence, non-maleficence, and justice, are well established as the basis of ethical practice for physicians.

Medical students are held to high standards of ethical behaviour; even actions taken outside of university can shape judgments about their fitness to practise (Turvill, 2015). There is, however, debate about how best to teach medical students to practise ethically. While some believe teaching ethical principles is enough, others argue that medical school must foster good character in physicians if they are to apply these principles in practice (Hafferty & Franks, 1994). Further, some have raised concern that medical school may produce poorer character in physicians through professional socialization that encourages physicians to become detached and less empathetic. While this chapter cannot address the entire debate about principlism, it is worth noting that discussion of ethical frameworks commonly associated with women are taking place in context of a wider debate about how best to practise ethically and to educate physicians to practise ethically.

There has also been debate about whether women and men differ in their capacity for moral reasoning. Much of this debate has centred around discussions of whether men and women make ethical decisions based on different principles or criteria. In the following sections, I outline two approaches to ethical decision making that have been seen as characteristically feminine or feminist. Although these overlap, I make a distinction between these two ethical frameworks to demonstrate the different ideas about gender that underlie them. The first, care ethics, is often described as a feminine approach to ethics. The second, feminist ethics, can be described as an approach to ethics that takes seriously gender-based power relations, in addition to other forms of oppression. While some feminists have taken inspiration from care ethics, this distinction helps to examine the implications of thinking about women physicians as distinctly different ethical decision makers.

Feminine Ethics of Care

Ethics of care is an approach to ethics that recognizes interdependence and caring relationships. Care ethicists argue that traditional approaches to ethics, such as principlism, centre traditionally masculine values such as justice, overlook the importance of caring motivation, and disregard context. Ethics of care is commonly associated with the work of Gilligan and Noddings. Gilligan (1982) countered previous work in moral psychology that suggested women are less capable of moral thought by arguing that women engage in a different (but not lesser) style of moral thinking. From Gilligan's (1982) perspective, women are more likely to draw on an ethic of care when they make moral decisions, and men are more likely to draw on an ethic of justice. In practice, this means that women are more likely to recognize individuals as interdependent, prioritize relationships, and act with empathy and compassion. Inspired by a maternal perspective, Noddings (1984) similarly centred caring relationships in her relational ethics. She argued that ethical principles cannot provide prescriptions for action. Instead, care must be applied in the context of a caring relationship.

These original versions of ethics of care have been criticized on a number of grounds. Three of these criticisms have significant relevance to the work of women physicians and will be discussed below. First, in lacking an explicit politics, care ethicists may ignore social structures, including the ways in which the burden of care work is distributed in society. Second, ethics of care perspectives may be essentialist in that they do not recognize differences between women. And third, ethics of care approaches offer few clear guidelines for action. Scholars continue to develop the ethics of care in ways that respond to these criticisms. Instead of conceptualizing care as a natural or essential moral practice of women, more recent versions of ethics of care involve a revaluation of caring as an approach to ethics that recognizes interdependence, values relationships, and encourages compassion. A collection edited by Held (1995) features more recent work in the ethics of care by Baier, Held, and Tronto.

Women Physicians as Ethical Careers?

Studies of patient assessments of physicians of different genders often demonstrate that women physicians are seen to be more empathetic or caring (Bylund & Makoul, 2002). Women physicians have been found to prioritize the caring relationship with patients by spending more time in consultations (Levinson & Lurie, 2004), developing collaborative relationships with their patients, and engaging patients in discussions of complex psychosocial issues (Heru, 2005). There is clearly an expectation that women physicians are more likely to be empathetic, compassionate, and nurturing in their practices.

From an ethics of care perspective, we could plausibly argue that women physicians are distinctly different in their ethical decision making because they prioritize care. This unique approach to ethical decision making may mean that women physicians are more likely to act on the principles of beneficence and non-maleficence, but may also make women less likely to make justice-based decisions required when not all patients can benefit. Although this is a plausible argument, I present a number of reasons to question the characterization of women physicians as ethical carers and consider the implications of viewing women physicians as distinctly different in their ethical practice because of their prioritization of care.

Methodologically, patient response surveys, which are often the basis for describing women physicians as more caring or empathetic, cannot often account for patients' gendered expectations or biases. Gendered expectations influence all of our social interactions. If a patient arrives to a clinical interaction assuming the woman physician is more caring than a man physician would be, this may lead the patient to share more personal information and express feelings more openly. In a meta-analysis, Hall and Roter (2002) found that patients communicate differently with female physicians by talking more and sharing more biomedical and psychosocial information. Berg and colleagues (2015) raise questions about gender biases in patient assessments of physician empathy. It remains unclear if women physicians actually demonstrate more empathy in practice, or if patients expect women physicians to be more empathetic and react differently based on this expectation.

Despite expressed preference for patient-centred care and belief that women physicians are more likely to be patient-centred, women physicians are barely preferred in patient surveys (Hall & Roter, 2002). Hall & Roter (2011) suggest three reasons for this disconnect. First, women physicians may be disadvantaged by the assumption that men are better physicians (Hall & Roter, 2011). Second, despite being more patient centred, women physicians may still breach gender stereotypes requiring women to be caring and approachable (Hall et al., 1994; Hall & Roter, 2011). Third, women physicians are in a double bind in which their communication style is seen as good female behaviour, not good physician behaviour (Blanch-Hartigan et al., 2010; Hall & Roter, 2011). Women physicians may not receive credit for their communication skills because it is expected of them to be caring and empathetic.

Further, assumptions that women physicians are more caring may lead to lower patient evaluations or criticism when individual physicians do not live up to this gendered ideal. Mast et al. (2008) found that satisfaction with female and male physicians is higher when physicians conformed to gender stereotypes. In other words, women physicians may be evaluated on how well they perform their role as women, not how well they perform their role as physicians. Women physicians are expected to be caring, nurturing, and empathetic because they are women. In this short chapter, women have been presented as a reasonably homogeneous social group. However, individual women have varied ways of performing their gender identities and these performances may adhere more or less to the gendered expectations discussed here. Gendered expectations of women physicians have serious implications for all women physicians, but may have more serious implications for women physicians who do not or cannot conform to these norms, including members of gender and sexual minority groups.

In practice, being seen as more caring in clinical interactions may increase the emotional labour required of women physicians. If patients are more likely to seek caring interactions with women physicians because of gendered expectations, women physicians will bear the burden of caring in health care systems. Studies have demonstrated that women physicians are likely to spend more time with patients (Levinson & Lurie, 2004) and that women physicians have reported high levels of stress (Stewart et al., 2000). This may be connected to the level of caring work they must engage in in their practices.

Further, the place of caring in medicine is often thought to be at the bedside or in family practice. From an ethical perspective, decisions made based on the ethics of care are often described as better for individual patients but not necessarily better for the health care system. Carers are thought to be less able to make justice-based decisions required by high-level administrators and medical educators. While there are increasing numbers of women physicians, high-level or powerful positions are still rarely held by women (Heru, 2005; Riska, 2001). If we argue that women are distinctly different in terms of their ethical decision making because they are more caring, we may further perpetuate the gendered expectations that keep women relegated to lower-level caring positions in the practice of medicine.

While it is seen as a compliment to suggest women physicians will humanize the profession, underlying assumptions about women as ethical carers limits women's advancement in the profession. Even in the context of gender socialization that encourages girls and women to be more nurturing, women physicians are not necessarily more caring and professional socialization may well counter gender socialization and limit differentiation between women and men physicians. Gendered expectations that women physicians are more caring may lead to the burden of more care work or poor evaluations by patients who expect a more nurturing provider.

Thus, arguing that women are distinctly different ethical decision makers because they prioritize caring over justice may be damaging to women physicians. That said, scholars have argued that revaluation of caring as an approach to ethics may be valuable. I agree with this assertion. Certainly, it would be valuable to reconsider the ways in which medical ethics training prioritizes "masculine" ethical principles over "feminine" ethical principles by recentring the caring roles of physicians. However, a revaluation of caring must occur profession-wide through changes in ethical training and expectations of all physicians. The burden of caring should not be placed on the shoulders of women physicians.

Feminist Ethics

Although often misunderstood or misused, feminism is an understanding that women are oppressed and a commitment to end this oppression. Oppression refers to the systematic and long-standing constraint of members of a social group based on their membership in that group (Frye, 1983). Recent work by feminists acknowledges the complex interactions between oppressions on the basis of gender, class, race, sexual orientation, and ability.

In contrast to what some call a "feminine" approach to ethics that prioritizes care, a feminist approach to ethics is political in the sense that "its ultimate aim is to identify and eliminate oppressive balances of power between people" (Tong, 1993, p. 160). Some feminist ethicists critique ethics of care perspectives for representing women as essentially different from men and lacking a political perspective (Sherwin, 1992). However, more recent work in the ethics of care may also be feminist (see for example, Baier et al. in Held, 1995).

The work of Sherwin (1992) and Tong (1993), and collections from Wolf (1996) and Anne Donchin and Laura Purdy (1999) provide good introductions and overviews of the field of feminist bioethics. Feminist bioethics shares with feminine care ethics recognition that individuals are interdependent and these relationships necessarily shape individuals. Feminist bioethics, however, is explicitly political in the sense that it requires examination of the ways in which social norms and power relations shape health and health care (Sherwin, 1992). In reference to health care practice, feminist bioethicists recognize the ways in which patient-provider interactions are structured by power relations and suggest ethical principles or practices be reimagined to account for these imbalances of power.

Women Physicians as Feminist Ethicists?

While most feminist scholars identify as women, it is not appropriate to suggest that women are "naturally" more inclined to have a feminist approach to ethical decision making. Unlike with ethics of care, girls and women are not often taught to be feminists through socialization. However, women's relative positions in social relations may provide a more readily available view of the oppressive power relations that constrain women (Harding, 1993). For example, women entering medicine may, because of their social experiences, have a better view of the ways in which medicine accepts male bodies as the norm in discussions of biology, the many ways in which men are seen as more skilled physicians, or how perceptions of women patients as less competent shapes their care. Although all women experience oppression, those women with the privilege to enter medical school may have significantly different social experiences than many other women and thus differing levels of knowledge of oppressive power relations.

Professional socialization may also quickly overcome social group differences and change women's perspectives on oppressive relations of power even if they entered training with these perspectives. There are few studies of the presence of feminist politics among medical students and physicians. Studies of medical socialization have demonstrated that medical training requires students leave behind their social group membership to become, as Beagan (2000) states, "neutral providers for (almost) neutral patients" (p. 53). Further, even those who maintain political views after medical school may not feel comfortable expressing them or acting on them for fear of appearing unprofessional. There is no evidence that women physicians are more likely to practise feminist ethics.

Women Physicians as Ethical Decision Makers

Both feminine and feminist approaches to ethics have been seen as distinctly women's approaches to ethics. However, there is little evidence that women physicians take a distinctly feminine or feminist approach to ethics. Gender socialization, gendered experiences, and gendered expectations may shape the ways in which women physicians perceive their role and their interactions with patients. This may, however, be diffused through professional socialization, which aims to produce neutral health care providers. If women physicians do approach ethical practice differently, whether through caring, recognition of power relations, or in another way, these approaches to ethical practice are not natural.

More broadly, we cannot assume that individuals entering medical school are naturally virtuous people who will practise ethically (Hafferty& Franks, 1994). Both revaluation of care (feminine ethics) and the integration of a political perspective into health care ethics (feminist ethics) provide important ways forward in the debate over how best to teach ethical practice and practise ethically. However, we cannot expect women physicians to have a distinctly different approach to ethics and, further, we cannot expect the addition of a large number of women physicians to change the culture of medical ethics.

Hopeful calls for women physicians to make medicine more caring and more responsive to the needs of patients suggest a need for widespread changes to ethical practice by health care providers. Significant changes in medical training, practice, and administration are required if feminine or feminist approaches to ethical practice are to be taken seriously. While women medical students may express more desire to learn about ethics and ethical practice (Roberts et al., 2004; Roberts et al., 2005), their relative positions of power within medicine limit the influence they may have (Heru, 2005; Riska, 2001).

Currently, detachment, objectivity, and impartiality are taught through a hidden curriculum in medical schools. The harsh treatment of medical students and residents, for example, counters efforts to teach caring and encourage empathy (Branch, 2000). Changes to ethical practice in medicine require explicit recognition of this hidden curriculum and introduction of a new ethics curriculum that encourages self-reflexivity, recognition of power structures that influence relationships and care provision, emotional engagement with patients, empathetic listening, and skills for self-care (among other skills). Distinct approaches to ethics often associated with women, feminine ethics, and feminist ethics, offer important ways forward in efforts to encourage ethical practice in health care settings. However, women physicians are not necessarily distinctly different in their ethical practice and the burden of humanizing medicine cannot and should not be placed on the shoulders of women physicians.

REFERENCES

Beagan, B.L. (2000, Oct). Neutralizing differences: Producing neutral doctors for (almost) neutral patients. *Social Science & Medicine (1982), 51*(8), 1253–65. https://doi.org/10.1016/S0277-9536(00)00043-5 Medline:11037215

Beauchamp, T.L., & Childress, J.F. (2001). *Principles of biomedical ethics* (5th ed.). New York: Oxford University Press.

Berg, K., Blatt, B., Lopreiato, J., Jung, J., Schaeffer, A., Heil, D., … Hojat, M. (2015, Jan). Standardized patient assessment of medical student empathy: Ethnicity and gender effects in a multi-institutional study. *Academic Medicine: Journal of the Association of American Medical Colleges, 90*(1), 105–11. https://doi.org/10.1097/ACM.0000000000000529 Medline:25558813

Biringer, A., & Carroll, J.C. (2012, Oct 16). What does the feminization of family medicine mean? *CMAJ, 184*(15), 1752. https://doi.org/10.1503/cmaj.120771 Medline:23008491

Blanch-Hartigan, D., Hall, J.A., Roter, D.L., & Frankel, R.M. (2010, Sep). Gender bias in patients' perceptions of patient-centered behaviors. *Patient Education and Counseling, 80*(3), 315–20. https://doi.org/10.1016/j.pec.2010.06.014 Medline:20638813

Branch, W.T., Jr., (2000, Feb). The ethics of caring and medical education. *Academic Medicine: Journal of the Association of American Medical Colleges, 75*(2), 127–32. https://doi.org/10.1097/00001888-200002000-00006 Medline:10693842

Bylund, C.L., & Makoul, G. (2002, Dec). Empathic communication and gender in the physician-patient encounter. *Patient Education and Counseling, 48*(3), 207–16. https://doi.org/10.1016/S0738-3991(02)00173-8 Medline:12477605

College of Family Physicians of Canada. (2010). 2010 national physician survey. Retrieved from http://nationalphysiciansurvey.ca/surveys/2010-survey/

de Beauvoir, S. (1972). *The second sex.* Harmondsworth, England: Penguin. (Originally published in 1949).

Donchin, A. & Purdy, L. (Eds.). (1999). *Embodying bioethics: Recent feminist advances*. New York: Rowman & Linfield.

Fausto-Sterling, A. (1992). Myths of gender: Biological theories about women and men. New York: Basic Books.

Frye, M. (1983). Oppression. In *The politics of reality: Essays in feminist theory* (pp. 1–16). New York: Crossing Press.

Gilligan, C. (1982). *In a different voice: Psychological theory and women's development*. Cambridge: Harvard University Press.

Hafferty, F.W., & Franks, R. (1994, Nov). The hidden curriculum, ethics teaching, and the structure of medical education. *Academic Medicine: Journal of the Association of American Medical Colleges*, *69*(11), 861–71. https://doi.org/10.1097/00001888-199411000-00001 Medline:7945681

Hall, J.A., Irish, J.T., Roter, D.L., Ehrlich, C.M., & Miller, L.H. (1994, Dec). Satisfaction, gender, and communication in medical visits. *Medical Care*, *32*(12), 1216–31. https://doi.org/10.1097/00005650-199412000-00005 Medline:7967860

Hall, J.A., & Roter, D.L. (2002, Dec). Do patients talk differently to male and female physicians? A meta-analytic review. *Patient Education and Counseling*, *48*(3), 217–24. https://doi.org/10.1016/S0738-3991(02)00174-X Medline:12477606

Hall, J.A., & Roter, D.L. (2011). Physician-patient communication. In H.S. Friedman (Ed.), *The Oxford handbook of health psychology* (pp. 317–46). New York: Oxford University Press.

Haraway, D. (1991). Situated knowledges. In D. Haraway (Ed.), *Simians, cyborgs, and women* (pp. 183–201). New York: Routledge.

Harding, S. (1993). Rethinking standpoint theory: What is strong objectivity? In L. Alcoff & E. Potter (Eds.), *Feminist epistemologies* (pp. 49–82). New York: Routledge.

Held, V. (1995). *Justice and care: Essential readings in feminist ethics*. Boulder, CO: Westview Press.

Herbert, C., Whiteside, C., McKnight, D., Verma, S., & Wilson, L. (2008, Mar 11). Ending the sexist blame game. *CMAJ*, *178*(6), 659, 661. https://doi.org/10.1503/cmaj.080216 Medline:18332373

Heru, A. (2005). Pink-collar medicine: Women and the future of medicine. *Gender Issues*, *22*(1), 20–34. https://doi.org/10.1007/s12147-005-0008-0

Levinson, W., & Lurie, N. (2004, Sep 21). When most doctors are women: what lies ahead? *Annals of Internal Medicine*, *141*(6), 471–4. https://doi.org/10.7326/0003-4819-141-6-200409210-00013 Medline:15381521

McKinstry, B., Colthart, I., Elliott, K., & Hunter, C. (2006, 05 10). The feminization of the medical work force, implications for Scottish primary care: a survey of Scottish general practitioners. *BMC Health Services Research*, *6*(1), 56. Retrieved from https://www.biomedcentral.com/1472-6963/6/56. https://doi.org/10.1186/1472-6963-6-56 Medline:16686957

Noddings, N. (1984). *Caring: A feminine approach to ethics and moral education*. Berkeley: University of California Press.

Pojman, L.P. (1990). *Discovering right and wrong*. Belmont, CA: Wadsworth Publishing Company.

Riska, E. (2001, Jan). Towards gender balance: but will women physicians have an impact on medicine? *Social Science & Medicine (1982)*, *52*(2), 179–87. https://doi.org/10.1016/S0277-9536(00)00218-5 Medline:11144774

Roberts, L.W., Green Hammond, K.A., Geppert, C.M.A., & Warner, T.D. (2004, Fall). The positive role of professionalism and ethics training in medical education: A comparison of medical student and resident perspectives. *Academic Psychiatry: The Journal of the American Association of Directors of Psychiatric Residency Training and the Association for Academic Psychiatry*, *28*(3), 170–82. https://doi.org/10.1176/appi.ap.28.3.170 Medline:15507551

Roberts, L.W., Warner, T.D., Hammond, K.A., Geppert, C.M.A., & Heinrich, T. (2005, Jul-Aug). Becoming a good doctor: perceived need for ethics training focused on practical and professional development topics. *Academic Psychiatry: The Journal of the American Association of Directors of Psychiatric Residency Training and the Association for Academic Psychiatry*, *29*(3), 301–9. https://doi.org/10.1176/appi.ap.29.3.301 Medline:16141129

Mast, M.S., Hall, J.A., Köckner, C., & Choi, E. (2008, Dec). Physician gender affects how physician nonverbal behavior is related to patient satisfaction. *Medical Care*, *46*(12), 1212–18. https://doi.org/10.1097/MLR.0b013e31817e1877 Medline:19300310

Sherwin, S. (1992). *No longer patient: Feminist ethics and health care*. Philadelphia: Temple University Press.

Stewart, D.E., Ahmad, F., Cheung, A.M., Bergman, B., & Dell, D.L. (2000, Mar). Women physicians and stress. *Journal of Women's Health & Gender-Based Medicine*, *9*(2), 185–90. https://doi.org/10.1089/152460900318687 Medline:10746522

Tong, R. (1993). *Feminine and feminist ethics*. Belmont, CA: Wadsworth Publishing Company.

Turvill, S. (2015). Common medicolegal problems faced by medical students: What legal support might you need as a medical student.*Student BMJ*, 23. Retrieved from http://student.bmj.com/student/view-article.html?id=sbmj.h168

Wolf, S.M. (1996). *Feminism and bioethics: Beyond reproduction*. New York: Oxford University.

10 Women and New Forms of Medicine

MONICA OLSEN, MAMTA GAUTAM, AND GILLIAN KERNAGHAN

Having led and facilitated many programs on aspects of leadership for medical women in the past 20 years, we have been struck by the depth of dialogue and sharing of vulnerabilities that women physicians demonstrate so readily. Women often come to these leadership development programs seeking to learn skills, and often do not give themselves credit for the skills they already have attained or the accomplishments they have already achieved. To set the stage as the workshops start, we typically ask participants who are currently in leadership roles to identify and share their joys and frustrations and for those moving into leadership roles to identify their hopes and fears. The following direct quotations from our workshop participants illustrate common themes and responses.

The common joys clearly reflect themes of benefits to oneself, benefits to others, and benefits to the system:

- "Living my values ... Making new positive professional connections when being authentic (heart-ful) self learning"
- "Seeing junior colleagues grow and develop ... connecting with others in a way that promotes meaningful growth ... being a mentor for a future leader ... seeing people being empowered"
- "Seeing end product success- meeting objectives, changing outcomes and improving health ... completing a project or difficult change"

The common frustrations are about impact to one's self, reactions from others, and systemic issues that do not support progress:

- "Too much to do and not enough me ... difficult role/too much conflict/ exhausting ... doing all the work and someone else takes the credit ... do I have time to do this?"

- "Surprising receipt of hostility … being undermined and bullied … resistance to change"
- "Getting down by process … bureaucratic bungling impedes process … glacial speed of change in most institutions … trying to change the culture"

The common hopes of new leaders are for what they can gain personally, what they can give to others, and how the system can be improved:

- "To become an effective leader within my clinical group without compromising my personal values and without belittling the contributions of others … personal enrichment while leading positive change … challenge myself … be seen as valuable"
- "Being an inspiration for others' growth … true collaboration – belief in a common goal … positive influence on incoming women leaders"
- "That I won't run out of time to influence the changes I want to see occur in medicine (education and overall delivery of care) … create meaningful change … provide direction … make a difference"

The common fears are primarily about fear of failure, which make up more than half the responses, concerns about work-life balance, and concern about perception of others:

- "Fear of failure - whatever that entails … letting perfect be the enemy of good"
- "Overcommitted and not meeting everyone's expectations … my ambitiousness overwhelms my personal life 'losing' in the work-life equation
- "Alienating colleagues … not being liked as much because now I'm the boss … being ineffective … being judged by my predecessors … being too nice … will anyone take me seriously?"

In these unedited words lies a profound need for these current and emerging women medical leaders to be true to themselves – to lead authentically. Authenticity, whereby people align their values and behaviours and are true to themselves, is a critical factor in leadership development. Researchers from the Center for Creative Leadership (CCL), highlight the importance of authenticity as "living a life strongly connected to your belief system promotes growth, learning and psychological well-being" (Ruderman & Rogolsky, 2014, p. 1). CCL research takes this further, stating that individual authenticity is crucial for organizations as well – those workplaces that nurture authentic behaviour have more engaged and productive workforces that are open and promote trust.

In this chapter, we will examine the current state of women in medicine and women leaders in medicine, and explore what women bring to leadership, both from the research and from our various interactions as facilitator, coach, psychiatrist, medical colleague, and medical leader.

The Current Reality of Women in Medicine

There are now more women in medicine than ever before. Major shifts in society during the 1960s and 1970s enabled women to access and participate in the workforce, and a parallel process has occurred in medicine too. First-year classes at medical schools across Canada first registered more women than men in 1997, and the numbers of female medical students and practicing physicians has been steadily rising since. The Canadian Medical Association projects that women will account for more than 45% of Canadian physicians by 2025. In 2014, women represented 38.1% of practicing physicians in Canada (Canadian Medical Association [CMA], 2015, p. 1). In the United States, there is a similar trend, as the percentage of female medical school graduates increased from 27% in 1983 to 48% in 2014 (Association of American Medical Colleges, 2014).

Specialty-specific patterns have been noted. Women represent 42.2% of physicians in family practice, as compared to 37.1% of medical specialists and 24.6% of surgical specialists (CMA, 2015). While there has been an increase in women residents in all specialties over the past 10 years, their career aspirations within medicine have remained remarkably similar. Women continue to gravitate to nonsurgical specialties and primary care, such as internal medicine, pediatrics, family practice, and OB-GYN.

The UK Royal College of Physicians (2009) summarized findings from its research into data on women in medicine in a document entitled *Women and Medicine: The Future*. It had two key findings, similar to those noted in North American studies. First, most women doctors have a preference for part-time or other flexible work. Second, women doctors showed a preference for working in specialties that offer more plannable working hours, and a relatively greater amount of patient interaction. It was suggested that both of these findings will affect future organization and delivery of health care, and the document made several recommendations for workforce design based on their findings.

Regardless of their choice of medical specialty, men and women practise differently in their clinical work and have differing practice styles. Studies have shown that in primary care, female physicians are more likely to deliver preventive services than their male colleagues, especially services for female patients, such as Pap smears for cancer screening (Bertakis et al., 1995; Franks & Clancy, 1993; Hall et al., 1990; Levy et al., 1992; Lurie et al., 1993; Osborn et al., 1991). There are differences among female and male physicians in their communication with patients. Female physicians are more likely to discuss concerns regarding lifestyle and social issues and offer more medical information to their patients (Elderkin-Thompson & Waitzkin, 1999; Hall et al., 1994; Meeuwesen et al., 1991; Roter & Hall, 1998; Roter et al., 1991). Female physicians were also more likely to have a participatory decision-making style in clinical care (Cooper-Patrick et al., 1999). In some studies, female physicians have been shown to spend more time with their patients than their male counterparts do (Bertakis & Robbins, 1987).

Williams and colleagues (1990) studied practice patterns and attitudes of women physicians in Canada. At that time, more women were entering medical school, and the impact of this increase was just starting to be felt in practice. Significant differences were noted in the organization and management of practices, as women preferred group practices and were overrepresented in community health centers and health service organizations. Only one-third of women, as compared to half the men, were in medical specialties. Even after adjusting for differences in workloads, incomes for women were significantly lower than for male colleagues.

In their book, Boulis and Jacobs (2008) drew upon hard data and anecdotes to analyse why so many women were entering medicine, how they fared once they became practicing physicians, and how they were transforming the way medicine is practised. They attributed women's entry into medicine less to the decline in the status of medicine and more to the changes within society regarding women's roles and options. They recognized existing disparities for women physicians concerning specialty choices, practice ownership, academic rank, leadership roles, and barriers to opportunity.

In 2013, a University of Montreal research team studied billing information of Quebec physicians, and concluded that the quality of care provided by female doctors was higher than that of their male counterparts, while the productivity of males is greater. Women physicians had significantly higher scores in compliance with practice guidelines. They were more likely than men to prescribe recommended medications and to plan required examinations. They were also more likely to earn significantly less than male colleagues (Borgès Da Silva et al., 2013).

Women in Medical Leadership Roles

Despite the increased entry of women into medicine, there remains an under-representation of women in leadership positions. The term *glass ceiling* has been used to describe an intangible yet real barrier to advancement within a profession, typically affecting women and minority groups. This is clearly no longer due to a pipeline effect whereby there are not enough qualified women heading down the pipeline towards leadership roles. Several studies have attempted to understand the barriers and make recommendations to address them. Some have argued that this is due to women physicians preferring to focus on their families over their careers. Women physicians do face challenges of combining work and family, as they temporarily leave work to start a family. They work fewer hours to spend more time at home when they have children, as they still bear the predominant responsibility for child care, which can be a barrier to career development (Schueller-Weidekamm & Kautzky-Willer, 2012). MacNamara et al. (2012) studied the lives of physician mothers, and showed that physician mothers were six times as likely to take care of their children after work hours compared to their partners/spouses. They identified other challenges they face, including the extensive length of training which may lead to delay in starting a family or fertility problems, double the emotional investment as they manage the responsibility for the health and well-being of others at work and at home, and a sense of balance between work and home responsibilities. Yet research shows that women are as interested as men to assume leadership roles, are equally qualified for the positions, and have equal leadership skills. Formal studies show that, in fact, women have more transformational and collaborative leadership styles, and may be more effective leaders than men (Eagly et al., 2003; Eagly & Karau, 2002).

Zhuge et al. (2011) confirmed that women were underrepresented as leaders in academic surgery. Women started their academic career with fewer resources, and tended to progress slower than men. They explore three main constraints for women leaders: traditional gender roles, which contribute to unconscious assumptions of abilities and negatively influence decisions regarding promotions; manifestations of sexism, both subtle and explicit, in the medical environment; and lack of effective mentors and role models that can lead to isolation and exclusion. Their article outlines strategies to address opportunities at both the individual and the institutional levels.

Kuhn et al. (2008) led a taskforce on women in academic emergency medicine that defined the current lack of women leaders; identified career barriers and potential solutions to recruitment, retention, and advancement; and created a document that made recommendations to improve the situation. They examined four levels of leadership: leadership of national emergency medicine organizations, medical school deans, department chairs, and individual women faculty members. For each level, they reviewed recommendations in the literature offered by national consensus groups and experts, and offered final recommendations reflecting the shared responsibility required to modify culture and address these issues.

Other studies confirm that gender-based differences in academic medical leadership exist. Sadeghpour et al. (2012) showed that sex-based differences in academic dermatology, including limitations for women regarding career track, academic rank distribution, leadership roles, and career satisfaction, persist. Based on a theory that women in academia are not selected for leadership because of low academic productivity, including fewer publications, Reed et al. (2011) compared publication records, academic promotions, and leadership roles for women physicians at Mayo Clinic. They found that women's publication rates increase and actually exceed those of men in the latter stages of their careers, yet women still hold fewer leadership positions. They suggest that academic productivity assessed at a midcareer point may not be an appropriate measure of leadership skills, and recommend that other factors be considered in selecting leaders. Marked gender disparities regarding top research leadership roles were also seen in the Department of Veterans Affairs, according to a study by (McCarren & Goldman, 2012)

There is concern that women leave academics at higher rates than men because of a lack of support. Levine et al. (2011) investigated possible reasons for women to leave academic medicine through structured individual interviews. A lack of role models for combining career and family responsibilities; frustrations with research, including funding difficulties, poor mentorship, and competition; desire for work-life balance; and an institutional environment described as non-collaborative and favouring male faculty all emerged as key factors that led to the decision to opt out of academic careers. The culture in medicine must be addressed to ensure that it provides the support and recognition required for success of women physicians. Recognizing that the work environment culture inhibits the career success of women in academic medicine, Westring et al. (2012) defined a construct of a culture conducive to women's academic success, which consisted of four distinct but related dimensions: equal access, work-life balance, freedom from gender biases, and supportive leadership. They also created a tool to measure the supportiveness of a culture and evaluate effectiveness of constructive interventions.

Thus, in 2015, gender parity had been realized among general practitioners; among specialists, we are closing the gap. However, there are unique issues for women in medicine as they deal with the competing demands of professional and personal lives, which impact how they practice. They bring a different approach and spend more time with each patient to communicate more and offer preventive measures. Inevitably, this change has an effect on the management of health care resources. As a profession, we need to prepare for these changes. Understanding now that women doctors tend to favour specific specialties and flexible working patterns will help medical schools create specialty training programs with this in mind, assist the government in health human resources planning, and help the profession to maintain the high standard of medical care in Canada. Women continue to achieve greater representation in academic medicine and leadership roles, although progress in these areas has been much slower. This, too, will need to be defined as we cannot afford the loss of such a large pool of talent and addressed to create a professional environment in which women physicians will succeed and advance.

The System Leadership Imperative

Canadians generally take pride in their health care system to the point that it is part of our national identity. It is a surprise to Canadians, and indeed to those who volunteer and work in the health care system in Canada, that we rank so low in the Commonwealth Fund ranking, coming in 10th out of 11 countries, with only the United States ranking lower (Davis et al., 2014). What is more concerning is that Canada ranks 9th out of 11 in both quality care and access and is the poorest performer in timeliness of care.

In contrast to these results are the patient satisfaction results that, for the most part, rank high in those aspects of the system where patient satisfaction is measured. Could it be that the expectations of patients are low, or is it that the individual care experience is generally good because of the care and attention of the people who serve in the system but not the system itself?

Health care at a provincial and territorial level consumes almost half of the governments' revenues. With the increased demands and expectations of the public, in addition to the aging population in most jurisdictions in Canada, there are considerable concerns regarding the sustainability of the health care system.

In August 2010, the CMA released a discussion document entitled *Health Care Transformation in Canada: Change That Works, Care That Lasts* (CMA, 2010). This was followed by a series of forums across Canada to engage Canadians in a broad discussion about the future of health care in Canada. In its summary document, the CMA stated "that there is a moral imperative to fix the system" (p. 34).

To fix the system, leadership will be required nationally, provincially and from all aspects of the system and from all contributors to the system. Canadian Health Leadership Network (CHLNet) recently published *Closing the Gap: A Canadian Health Leadership Action Plan* (2014). In the action plan, the results of a recent CHLNet benchmarking study are highlighted, showing 84% of health care leaders are concerned about the overall leadership gap, with 42% of Canadian Academic Health Sciences Centres reporting they do not have the leadership they need to meet the challenges of the future.

The action plan speaks to essential components of leadership to contribute to health system transformation. A key component is a collective vision of what we are trying to create. There is limited opportunity to achieve this at a national level, given the provincial accountability for health care. In addition, the political aspect of health care can make a sustainable vision a challenge at times.

Another key component of the action plan is a common leadership platform. LEADS in a Caring Environment is a common leadership platform that has organically spread across the country and is used in health care organizations, national leadership organizations, and professional organizations (Dickson & Tholl, 2011). LEADS is a framework of leadership capabilities and competencies that features five domains: lead self, engage others, achieve results, develop coalitions, and systems transformation. Each of these five domains consists of four core, measurable capabilities. Indeed, the CMA, in partnership with the Canadian Society of Physician Leaders, has adopted LEADS as the measure by which applicants for the Canadian Certified Physician Executive credential will be evaluated.

In a report entitled *Exploring the Dynamics of Physician Engagement and Leadership for Health System Improvement* (Denis et al., 2013), the authors' first key message is that "physician leadership and physician engagement are essential elements of high-performing healthcare systems, contributing to higher scores on many quality indicators" (p. 1).

Transformational change requires new strategies, generally organization or system wide, over time to achieve the desired outcomes. Transformational leaders are individuals who identify the needed change, define a vision and are able to inspire others to work together to achieve the vision.

Given the fact that women now account for half of the medical school graduates, it will be imperative for female physicians to prepare for and engage in health care system leadership if we are going to transform the system.

Does a Distinct Female Leadership Style Exist?

In their 2007 article "Women and the Labyrinth of Leadership," Alice Eagly and Linda Carli (2007) referenced a meta-analysis which integrated the results of 45 studies addressing the question, "Does a distinct female leadership style exist?"

In this research, Eagly (2007) devised and used a framework that distinguishes between transformational and transactional leadership. In brief, transformational leaders

- demonstrate qualities that motivate respect and pride from association with them (positive role modelling by gaining followers' trust and confidence)
- exhibit optimism and excitement about goals and future states
- examine new perspectives for solving problems and completing tasks
- state future goals, develop plans to achieve those goals, and innovate even if the organization is successful
- mentor and empower followers to develop their full potential

By contrast, transactional leaders

- provide rewards for satisfactory performance by followers
- attend to followers' mistakes and failures to meet standards
- wait until problems become severe before attending to them and intervening

Although most leaders embrace some behaviours from both types, the researchers also allowed for a third category, called the laissez-faire style – a style characterized by frequent absence and lack of involvement during critical moments.

"The meta-analysis found in general female leaders were somewhat more transformational than male leaders, especially when it came to giving support and encouragement to subordinates. They also engaged in more of the rewarding behaviours that are one aspect of transactional leadership" (Eagly & Carli, 2007, p. 9). Men exceeded women on the transactional leadership aspects involving corrective and disciplinary actions and were also more likely to be laissez-faire leaders.

Given that most leadership research has extolled the benefits of the transformational style (along with the rewards and positive incentives associated with the transactional style) for today's organizations, the research suggests "women's approaches are more generally effective – while men's often are only somewhat effective or actually hinder effectiveness." (Eagly & Carli, 2007, p. 9). In a separate meta-analysis, women were found to adopt a more participative and collaborative style than men typically favour. A possible interpretation for this is that collaboration can get results without appearing to be masculine or autocratic, which followers may find objectionable in female leaders.

Transformational leadership was first introduced as a concept by James McGregor Burns in 1978. He defined it as leadership where the "leaders and their followers raise one another to higher levels of morality and motivation" (Burns, 1978). Burns's work was further developed by Bernard M Bass (1990), who spoke of transformational leadership as leadership in which both leadership and performance are beyond expectations. Transformational leaders are generally passionate and enthusiastic, motivating others to be their best in achieving the desired outcomes through a shared vision. In Eagly's summary (2007), she identifies differences in female and male leadership styles but the evidence of better outcomes based on a predominant male or female leadership style is lacking. Male and female physicians need to work together in leadership to bring about the transformational change required in health care today.

Developing Leaders

Leaders are developed much like physicians are developed – through academic preparation, experience, coaching, mentoring, and sponsorship. There is needed academic preparation, providing foundational knowledge about system and leadership styles, capabilities, and competencies. Although women may be more transformational in their leadership style, these styles need to adapt to team, organizational, or system needs. Leaders who are able to adapt will be more successful in this complex system called health care.

Leaders are also developed through experience, when they take the opportunity to lead and view this role, formal or informal, as a learning experience. Think about how more positive our approach to joining or chairing a committee would be if we could grasp the learning we will gain rather than seeing it as a burden.

In Ontario, the *Public Hospitals Act* defines a medical staff organization as an organization within a hospital that represents physicians in their relationship with the hospital. The president of the medical staff organization has an ex officio seat on the board of directors. It has been a challenge in recent years in many hospitals to attract physicians to serve their colleagues in this. However, for a limited time commitment, the person in this role will have a seat on the board, learning the difference between governance and management. He or she will also learn the complexity of the hospital system as it relates to the interface between quality of care and the work environment and funding. In addition, this person will learn about capital versus operating funding and the obligations on the organization related to multiple pieces of legislation. One key opportunity gained by serving on a hospital board is to work with passionate and committed community volunteers who give generously of their time for the betterment of their community's health care. This same opportunity could be described for many of the committees and initiatives in which physicians have the chance to be engaged.

The third component of the development of leaders is in coaching, mentoring, or sponsorship. Kathy Hopinkah Hannan (2015), a national managing partner at KPMG LLP US, who has shattered the glass ceiling in a traditionally male-dominated field of accounting, shares her firsthand knowledge of what it takes to succeed, and clarifies the difference: "A mentor is someone who speaks *with* you.... A coach speaks *to* you.... A sponsor will speak *for* you."

Increasingly, physician leaders are engaging executive coaches, and some physicians are becoming trained as coaches themselves. Some coaches are paid for by the physicians themselves or by their organizations. Coaching used to be seen as a way to help underperforming individuals develop; however, in recent years, coaching has increasingly focused on the development of individuals' job performance for those who are seen as future executive leaders. Coaching should mainly focus on the development of strengths, with less focus on weaknesses.

Mentorship has been established more in academic medicine domains to support new physician faculty in their academic careers. A mentor is a more experienced person in your field who offers you counsel, guidance, and career advice. Many physicians have experienced the value of having a person who can assist them with real life experiences in their career development.

Sponsorship has been more ingrained in the corporate world and may have value in academic medicine or other health care organizations. In an article in *Academic Medicine*, "Sponsorship: A Path to the Academic Medicine C-suite for Women Faculty" (Travis et al., 2013), the authors define sponsorship as that public support by a powerful, influential person for the advancement and promotion of an individual within whom the sponsor sees untapped or unappreciated leadership talent or potential. The authors speak to the value of this in the corporate world, which has supported the development of female leaders and positioned them to earn top executive positions with merit.

Female physicians are taking on many leadership roles within the health care system, from lead physician in a clinic to CEO of large organizations. When women complete their medical training, many are thinking of starting a family. Balancing a busy medical career with family can be challenging. Female physicians who also aspire to leadership are, at times, discouraged from taking on leadership roles early in their career while trying to find work-life balance.

Possible Concerns for Women Leaders

In their book *The Confidence Code: The Science and Art of Self-Assurance – What Women Should Know*, Kay and Shipman (2014) discuss several prevailing beliefs that women hold about themselves. They identify a key belief held by women is that they simply do not believe they are good enough. Other critical findings explored in the book reveal that, in contrast to men, women have a much higher fear of failure, are more risk–adverse, and ruminate on elements that they have done wrong for significantly longer – all contributing to the erosion of confidence and, consequently, to inaction. This was in keeping with our findings based on questions asked at the start of workshops for women leaders in medicine.

As if that were not enough, the authors also provide research that shows that women are 25% more prone to perfectionism than men (Kay & Shipman, 2014). This pursuit of perfection may set up a vicious cycle beginning with unrealistic self-expectations, followed by self-blame for inevitably poor results, leading to procrastination, lowered confidence, or defensiveness, then potentially to reduced productivity, and ultimately to a repeat of unrealistic expectations, demanding even higher standards. Given that it is generally accepted that academia and medicine tend to draw perfectionists, women need to be even more alert to this potential unhealthy cycle.

Another related dynamic that women need to be alert to is the "imposter phenomenon" (Clance & Imes, 1978, p. 1). Essentially this "label" describes the self-doubt that many people, particularly high achievers, experience. Basically, it is a sense that you do not really know what you are doing and that you have fooled others into believing that you are more competent and talented than you really are. Consequences and implications of this phenomenon may include experiencing anxiety, being uncomfortable with praise, avoiding asking relevant questions, seeking appropriate help for assigned work, avoiding growth opportunities, speaking one's mind assertively or burdening oneself with too much work to compensate for lack of self-esteem ("just not good enough") and identity ("could do better if only they worked harder") (Clance & Imes, 1978, p. 1).

Women are more prone to the imposter phenomenon for three reasons: (1) gender role socialization, especially at critical junctures (e.g., marriage, work, and children); (2) functioning in a male dominated environment where competitive male colleagues assume something other than talent or skill was responsible for success; or (3) many women are not aware of their talents, and if they are, they are more likely to hide those talents to deal with others' envy and their own feelings of self-doubt.

In light of the proliferation of this phenomenon and the restraint it poses on personal and professional fulfilment, and its negative impact on engagement, it is critical to overcome this problem. Recommendations on this subject would involve awareness and education on this topic, strengths-based practices in curriculums and organization cultures, and research focused on organizational engagement strategies to help identify and address this issue.

There are, however, many examples of female physician leaders who have successfully integrated leadership careers, clinical practice, and personal life. It is incumbent on those female physicians who have traversed this journey to act as mentors and sponsors to younger female colleagues.

Another important aspect of leadership is the context in which one is leading. This is what we refer to as "system literacy." In medical school, there is limited or no exposure to the system in which we work clinically or academically. There are important aspects that we are never taught, such as how it is funded, how decisions are made, what the legislative framework and regulations are, and how it is governed. This is key knowledge for formal or informal physician leaders to facilitate constructive engagement with other system leaders.

Are all physicians leaders? Many physicians assume informal leadership roles in a team or in a clinic. As such, it is vitally important that physicians develop some capability in the first three aspects of the LEADS framework (Dickson & Tholl, 2011), which are leading self, engaging others and achieving results. Emotional intelligence is foundational in the first two capabilities.

From the Research on Emotional and Social Intelligence

"Look deeply at almost any factor that influences organizational effectiveness, and you will find that emotional intelligence plays a role" was fittingly stated by (Cherniss & Goleman, 2001, p. 4). Since 2001, we have seen a proliferation of leadership development programs that have embedded emotional intelligence (EI) into their curriculums and capabilities framework, including the Canadian LEADS in Caring Environment Capabilities Framework (Dickson & Tholl, 2011), thereby moving beyond the traditional business acumen and technical aptitude requirements. It is now more clearly recognized that leaders are in pivotal roles to shape organizational culture and, ultimately, to impact an organization's performance. It behooves us to examine this new type of intelligence edge and determine how it fits with the natural strengths that women bring to leadership roles, in light of the increasing demographic shift of women in medicine. Layered with this is the fact that developing the next generation of leaders is a looming concern, given the exit of baby boomers.

One of the authors (Monica Olsen) has worked in the field of organization effectiveness for over 25 years, primarily in the area of leadership development in health care. This experience has provided her with immensely satisfying opportunities to administer hundreds of emotional intelligence assessments and feedback debrief sessions. She has used the BarOn EQ-i assessment, the world's first scientifically validated instrument and the subsequent Emotional Quotient Inventory 2.0, a popular EI measurement based on the Bar-On EQ-i model by (Bar-On & Parker, 2000). She has additionally facilitated EI programs for health care leaders at various experience levels, as well as open and intact work groups.

Research conducted by Multi-Health Systems (MHS), a leading publisher of psychological assessments in the area of emotional intelligence among others, recently led to its EQ-i 2.0 leadership report. In its leadership sample data collection, MHS demonstrated that leaders score significantly higher in EI than the general population (North American norm group). Furthermore, results indicated that those with predominantly *transformational* leadership styles scored significantly higher than those with predominantly *transactional* leadership styles (MHS Website EQ-I 2.0 Leadership Report Interpretive Guide). Of even more interest is that transformational leaders also had substantially higher scores (ds > .2) on virtually all the subscales with the exceptions being assertiveness, independence, and problem-solving, the last two of which men usually scored higher on as noted by Bar-On in his earlier normative sample (Bar-On & Parker, 2000, p. 367). This may suggest that male leaders have a preference for transactional leadership styles. We have previously stated the clear need for transformational leadership to effectively affect system change in health care.

Although women and men (Bar-On & Parker, 2000) score similarly in their overall emotional and social competence, significant gender differences do exist for some factors (Bar-On & Parker, 2000, p. 367). Females appear to have stronger interpersonal skills than males, more specifically, women are more aware of emotions, demonstrate more empathy, relate better interpersonally, and act more socially responsible than men. From an EI perspective, it may well appear that women leaders are more poised for transformational leadership styles. Men's score differences showed up as higher in self-regard, independence, stress tolerance, flexibility, problem-solving, and optimism than women, which may well lend to a preferred transactional style of leadership.

From the EQ-i assessment debrief sessions with physicians, I have noticed a trend of higher scores in empathy and social responsibility with women medical leaders compared to their male colleagues. What stands out as trends in the lower score range are self-regard and assertiveness among this group compared to their male colleagues. Often, discussions among medical women leaders focus on the women feeling like "imposters," the dynamic described earlier in this chapter. Clearly, more research is required to determine those factors that erode/impact self-regard and assertiveness, and to explore how to more effectively balance the higher scores of empathy and social responsibility found in women's assessments.

What Women Bring to Leadership

Having briefly looked at the EI traits that women bring to their roles, we will now look at other compelling traits that women bring to leadership. There is a growing body of research that shows a driver for engaging with people is to provide meaningful work experiences that leverage their strengths. What role do organization leaders play in building their leadership talent capacity? What role could they play?

In a recent study of more than 25,000 Harvard Business School MBA graduates (Ely et al., 2014), across three generations from baby boomers to millennials, the researchers were interested in learning what was contributing to gender gaps in business and other sectors. There is value in looking at this research, as there are parallels between this study group and highly educated, career-oriented physicians when it comes to prevailing beliefs and possible strategies.

One common belief as to why high-potential women quit their jobs was to care for their families (Ely et al., 2014). In fact, the majority who did quit went on to other jobs and did not stay home to care for children. They leave if they find themselves in unfulfilling roles with dim prospects for growth or advancement. The authors identified that further research was needed on how professional men and women navigate their family and career decisions, and the impact that family responsibilities have on both women and men's careers. Traditional partnerships were linked to higher career satisfaction for men, whereas women who ended up in such arrangements were less satisfied, regardless of original expectations. Those women whose careers and child care responsibilities were seen as equal to their partners were as satisfied as the men. As millennials begin their families, it remains to be seen how mismatched (partner) expectations will play out. Another myth that needs to be addressed is that women value career less than men, or that mothers do not want high-profile, challenging work. The reality for this study group is that they value both fulfilment at work and life outside of work. Organizations need to move beyond current arrangements and policies to be family-friendly. Women want more meaningful work and more opportunities for career growth. Otherwise, if this is not available and they feel that their careers are stalling, they may default to a support role in which their jobs are secondary.

Final Thoughts

Women constitute an increasing number of physicians in Canada. There are noted differences from their male colleagues in their choice of specialty, practice patterns, and communication styles. While the numbers of women in medicine have increased, they are not proportionately represented in medical leadership roles. There is a system imperative requiring physicians to step up as leaders if we are collectively going to improve the quality, performance and sustainability of health care in Canada. Male and female leaders bring unique strengths to leadership. Such diversity is positive and will serve to enrich the strategic dialogue and subsequent actions required to achieve the quality health care system that the Canadian population desires and believes they have.

REFERENCES

Association of American Medical Colleges. (2014). Table 1: Chart 4: US medical school applications and matriculants by school, state of legal residence and sex. Retrieved from https://www.aamc.org/data/facts/

Bar-On, R., & Parker, J. (2000). *The handbook of emotional intelligence, theory, development, assessment and application at home, school, and in the workplace.* San Francisco: Jossey-Bass/Wiley.

Bass, B.M. (1990). From transactional to transformational leadership: Learning to share the vision. *Organizational Dynamics, 18*(3), 19–31.

Bertakis, K.D., & Robbins, J.A. (1987, Mar). Gatekeeping in primary care: A comparison of internal medicine and family practice. *The Journal of Family Practice, 24*(3), 305–9. Medline:3819670

Bertakis, K.D., Helms, L.J., Callahan, E.J., Azari, R., & Robbins, J.A. (1995, Apr). The influence of gender on physician practice style. *Medical Care, 33*(4), 407–16. https://doi.org/10.1097/00005650-199504000-00007 Medline:7731281

Borgès Da Silva, R., Martel, V., & Blais, R. (2013). Qualité et productivité dans les groupes de médecine de famille: qui sont les meilleurs? Les hommes ou les femmes?*Revue d'Épidémiologie et de Santé Publique, 61*(Suppl 4), S210–S211.

Boulis, A.K., & Jacobs, J.A. (2008). *The changing face of medicine: Women doctors and the evolution of health care in America*. Ithaca, NY: ILR Press Book.

Burns, J.M. (1978). *Leadership*. New York: Harper and Row.

Canadian Health Leadership Network. (2014). Closing the gap: A Canadian health leadership action plan. Retrieved from https://www.cchl-ccls.ca/document/1126/CHLNet_CanadianHealthLeadershipActionPlan.pdf.

Canadian Medical Association. (2010). Healthcare transformation in Canada: Change that works, care that lasts. Retrieved from http://policybase.cma.ca/dbtw-wpd/PolicyPDF/PD10-05.PDF

Canadian Medical Association. (2015). Number and percent distribution of physicians by specialty and sex, Canada 2015. Retrieved from https://www.cma.ca/Assets/assets-library/document/en/advocacy/06SpecSex.pdf

Chernise & Goleman, D. (2001). *The emotionally intelligent workplace*. San Francisco: Jossey-Bass.

Cooper-Patrick, L., Gallo, J.J., Gonzales, J.J., Vu, H.T., Powe, N.R., Nelson, C., & Ford, D.E. (1999, Aug 11). Race, gender, and partnership in the patient-physician relationship. *JAMA, 282*(6), 583–9. https://doi.org/10.1001/jama.282.6.583 Medline:10450723

Clance, P.R., & Imes, S. (1978). The imposter phenomenon in high achieving women: Dynamics and therapeutic intervention. *Psychotherapy (Chicago, Ill.), 15*(3), 241–7. https://doi.org/10.1037/h0086006

Davis, K., Stremikis, K., Squires, D., & Schoen, C. (2014). *Mirror, mirror on the wall: How the performance of the U.S. health care system compares internationally*. New York: Commonwealth Fund. Retrieved from http://www.commonwealthfund.org/~/media/files/publications/fund-report/2014/jun/1755_davis_mirror_mirror_2014.pdf

Denis, J.-L., Baker, G.R., Black, C., Langley, A., Lawless, B., Leblanc, D., Lusiani, M., Hepburn, C.M., Pomey, M.-P., & Tré, G. (2013). Exploring the dynamics of physician engagement and leadership for health system improvement: Prospects for Canadian healthcare systems. Retrieved from http://www.cfhi-fcass.ca/SearchResultsNews/13-04-16/c2dcf12c-680f-4b63-91ab-bc3e726b523f.aspx

Dickson, G., & Tholl, B. (2011). *LEADS in a caring environment capabilities framework.* Retrieved from http://www.hqontario.ca/Portals/0/modals/qi/en/processmap_pdfs/resources_links/leads%20handout%20(jan%202012).pdf

Eagly, A. (2007). Female leadership advantage & disadvantage: Resolving the contradictions. *Psychology of Women Quarterly, 31*(1), 1–12. https://doi.org/10.1111/j.1471-6402.2007.00326.x

Eagly, A.H., & Carli, L.L. (2007, Sep). Women and the labyrinth of leadership. *Harvard Business Review, 85*(9), 62–71, 146. Medline:17886484

Eagly, A.H., Johannesen-Schmidt, M.C., & van Engen, M.L. (2003, Jul). Transformational, transactional, and laissez-faire leadership styles: a meta-analysis comparing women and men. *Psychological Bulletin, 129*(4), 569–91. https://doi.org/10.1037/0033-2909.129.4.569 Medline:12848221

Eagly, A.H., & Karau, S.J. (2002, Jul). Role congruity theory of prejudice toward female leaders. *Psychological Review, 109*(3), 573–98. https://doi.org/10.1037/0033-295X.109.3.573 Medline:12088246

Ely, R.J., Stone, P., & Ammerman, C. (2014). Rethink what you "know" about high-achieving women. *Harvard Business Review.* Retrieved from https://hbr.org/2014/12/rethink-what-you-know-about-high-achieving-women

Elderkin-Thompson, V., & Waitzkin, H. (1999, Feb). Differences in clinical communication by gender. *Journal of General Internal Medicine, 14*(2), 112–21. https://doi.org/10.1046/j.1525-1497.1999.00296.x Medline:10051782

Franks, P., & Clancy, C.M. (1993, Mar). Physician gender bias in clinical decision making: screening for cancer in primary care. *Medical Care, 31*(3), 213–218. https://doi.org/10.1097/00005650-199303000-00003 Medline:8450679

Hall, J.A., Palmer, R.H., Orav, E.J., Hargraves, J.L., Wright, E.A., & Louis, T.A. (1990, Jun). Performance quality, gender, and professional role: A study of physicians and nonphysicians in 16 ambulatory care practices. *Medical Care, 28*(6), 489–501. https://doi.org/10.1097/00005650-199006000-00002 Medline:2355755

Hall, J.A., Irish, J.T., Roter, D.L., Ehrlich, C.M., & Miller, L.H. (1994, Dec). Satisfaction, gender, and communication in medical visits. *Medical Care, 32*(12), 1216–31. https://doi.org/10.1097/00005650-199412000-00005 Medline:7967860

Hannan, K. (2015, May 20). Why you are never too old to have a mentor. *Fortune.* Retrieved from http://fortune.com/2015/05/20/kathy-hannan-importance-of-a-mentor

Kay, K., & Shipman, C. (2014). *The confidence code: The science and art of self-assurance – What women should know.* New York: Harper-Business.

Kuhn, G.J., Abbuhl, S.B., Clem, K.J., & Society for Academic Emergency Medicine (SAEM) taskforce for women in academic emergency medicine. (2008, Aug). Recommendations from the Society for Academic Emergency Medicine (SAEM) Taskforce on women in academic emergency medicine. *Academic Emergency Medicine: Official Journal of the Society for Academic Emergency Medicine, 15*(8), 762–7. https://doi.org/10.1111/j.1553-2712.2008.00190.x Medline:18783488

Levine, R.B., Lin, F., Kern, D.E., Wright, S.M., & Carrese, J. (2011, Jun). Stories from early-career women physicians who have left academic medicine: A qualitative study at a single institution. *Academic Medicine: Journal of the Association of American Medical Colleges, 86*(6), 752–8. https://doi.org/10.1097/ACM.0b013e318217e83b Medline:21512363

Levy, S., Dowling, P., Boult, L., Monroe, A., & McQuade, W. (1992, Jan). The effect of physician and patient gender on preventive medicine practices in patients older than fifty. *Family Medicine, 24*(1), 58–61. Medline:1520350

Lurie, N., Slater, J., McGovern, P., Ekstrum, J., Quam, L., & Margolis, K. (1993, Aug 12). Preventive care for women: Does the sex of the physician matter? *The New England Journal of Medicine, 329*(7), 478–82. https://doi.org/10.1056/NEJM199308123290707 Medline:8332153

MacNamara, M.M., Taylor, J.S., Grimm, K.J., Taylor, L.E., & Gottlieb, A.S. (2012, Jun). Using a professional organization, MomDocFamily, to understand the lives of physician-mothers. *Medicine and Health, Rhode Island, 95*(6), 189–93. Medline:22866508

McCarren, M., & Goldman, S. (2012, Aug). Research leadership and investigators: gender distribution in the federal government. *The American Journal of Medicine, 125*(8), 811–16. https://doi.org/10.1016/j.amjmed.2012.03.006 Medline:22579138

Meeuwesen, L., Schaap, C., & van der Staak, C. (1991). Verbal analysis of doctor-patient communication. *Social Science & Medicine (1982), 32*(10), 1143–50. https://doi.org/10.1016/0277-9536(91)90091-P Medline:2068597

Osborn, E.H., Bird, J.A., McPhee, S.J., Rodnick, J.E., & Fordham, D. (1991, May). Cancer screening by primary care physicians: Can we explain the differences? *The Journal of Family Practice, 32*(5), 465–71. Medline:2022934

Public Hospitals Act, RSO 1990, c P.40. Retrieved from http://www.ontario.ca/laws/regulation/900965

Reed, D.A., Enders, F., Lindor, R., McClees, M., & Lindor, K.D. (2011, Jan). Gender differences in academic productivity and leadership appointments of physicians throughout academic careers. *Academic Medicine: Journal of the*

Association of American Medical Colleges, 86(1), 43–7. https://doi.org/10.1097/ACM.0b013e3181ff9ff2 Medline:21099390

Roter, D., Lipkin, M., Jr., & Korsgaard, A. (1991, Nov). Sex differences in patients' and physicians' communication during primary care medical visits. *Medical Care, 29*(11), 1083–93. https://doi.org/10.1097/00005650-199111000-00002 Medline:1943269

Roter, D.L., & Hall, J.A. (1998, Nov). Why physician gender matters in shaping the physician-patient relationship. *Journal of Women's Health, 7*(9), 1093–7. https://doi.org/10.1089/jwh.1998.7.1093 Medline:9861586

Royal College of Physicians. (2009). Women and medicine: The future. Summary of findings from Royal College of Physicians research. London: Author.

Ruderman, M., & Rogolsky, S. (2014). Getting real: How high-achieving women can lead authentically. Center for Creative Leadership White Paper. Retrieved from https://www.ccl.org/wp-content/uploads/2015/04/GettingReal.pdf

Sadeghpour, M., Bernstein, I., Ko, C., & Jacobe, H. (2012, Jul). Role of sex in academic dermatology: Results from a national survey. *Archives of Dermatology, 148*(7), 809–14. https://doi.org/10.1001/archdermatol.2011.3617 Medline:22801614

Schueller-Weidekamm, C., & Kautzky-Willer, A. (2012, Aug). Challenges of work-life balance for women physicians/mothers working in leadership positions. *Gender Medicine, 9*(4), 244–50. https://doi.org/10.1016/j.genm.2012.04.002 Medline:22626768

Travis, E.L., Doty, L., & Helitzer, D.L. (2013, Oct). Sponsorship: A path to the academic medicine C-suite for women faculty? *Academic Medicine: Journal of the Association of American Medical Colleges, 88*(10), 1414–17. https://doi.org/10.1097/ACM.0b013e3182a35456 Medline:23969365

Westring, A.F., Speck, R.M., Sammel, M.D., Scott, P., Tuton, L.W., Grisso, J.A., & Abbuhl, S. (2012, Nov). A culture conducive to women's academic success: development of a measure. *Academic Medicine: Journal of the Association of American Medical Colleges, 87*(11), 1622–31. https://doi.org/10.1097/ACM.0b013e31826dbfd1 Medline:23018337

Williams, A.P., Domnick-Pierre, K., Vayda, E., Stevenson, H.M., & Burke, M. (1990, Aug 1). Women in medicine: Practice patterns and attitudes. *CMAJ, 143*(3), 194–201. Medline:2379127

Zhuge, Y., Kaufman, J., Simeone, D.M., Chen, H., & Velazquez, O.C. (2011, Apr). Is there still a glass ceiling for women in academic surgery? *Annals of Surgery, 253*(4), 637–43. Medline:21475000

11 Patients, Women Family Doctors, and Patient-Centred Care

PERLE FELDMAN

I am a liminal person. My career has spanned the time from when women were rare in medicine to now, when they are the majority of students in almost every faculty of medicine in Canada and in many specialties.

The year before I started medical school in 1976, there were 10 women in the class of 160 students. This number had been consistent for years. These women were the magnificent exceptions, brilliant, driven, and often marginalized. Our class, in contrast, had 60 women. The University, and certainly the hospitals, were not ready for this monstrous regiment of women. When we started small groups in second year it was not unusual for our preceptors to walk into a room and see six women and four men, all freshly scrubbed in our short white coats, our pockets bulging with equipment, and turn around and say, "Oh, sorry, I was looking for the medical students." The Royal Victoria Hospital had exactly four beds for female clerks in 1978, and some nights we slept tag-team, one of us taking the warm and fragrant spot of another student who had just been called out, or curling up in a lounge with a flannel blanket and spare pillow donated by a charitable nurse.

The patients were also suspicious then. I had patients refuse me, because they wanted "a man doctor, a real doctor." My preceptors felt the need to assure patients that the three young women in our internal medicine group were really medical students and were allowed to examine them. I know that the day the male head nurse on the medical floor introduced me to a patient as "the young doctor who will be caring for you," the patient's head bounced back and forth in disbelief. This picture of the nurse as a man and the doctor as a woman was something completely new and unbelievable in his reality.

I remember a patient, a man in his fifties, making a pass at me. Even though I was shocked and dismayed I understood that at some level he could only process a woman taking an interest in him and touching him as a sexual act.

Nowadays, this expectation is reversed and many, if not most, patients prefer a woman physician, particularly in primary care. However, when people say to me that they think women doctors are better than the men I often think that this is a kind of old-fashioned attitude. When there were only eight to ten women in any medical school class, of course they were brilliant and exceptional in every way. That was the only way they got in. This is similar to the now largely forgotten belief that Jewish doctors were better, and for the same reason. The quotas of the 1940s to 1950s almost guaranteed that those who got through that restrictive selection criteria were better than those who faced fewer obstacles.

One of my earliest mentors, Dr Mary Ellen Kirk, a brilliant pathologist, told me that one of the reasons she had decided not to do clinical medicine was that she felt the patients who went to women physicians, in her day, were a particular cohort. She thought they were needier, whinier, and much more likely to be somatizers. I don't know if that was true but she was not the only one with that perception.

When I began my own practice in 1985, I took over from a man who left to go on to do infectious disease training. Within a few weeks my secretary commented that I spent a lot more time with my patients than he did. I also seemed to write significantly fewer benzodiazepine prescriptions than he did. These were not independent phenomena.

In the literature it is known that women physicians tend to spend more time with their patients. The difference is significant although small. The length of visit averaged 21 min (range 7.4–36.7 min) for male physicians and 23 min (range 10.5–37 min) for female physicians (Hall et al., 2015). In the extra time they engage in more patient-centred communications. They ask more questions, make more empathic statements, and give more biomedical and psychosocial information. Their patients talk more, so the encounters are more interactive (Hall et al., 2015).

We know that female family doctors do more screening than their male counterparts (Dollin, 2002). It was believed that this was because they have a higher proportion of female patients with increased need for women's health screening, such as mammograms and pap tests. However, a paper by Henderson & Weisman (2001) showed that female physicians did more screening and counselling than their male counterparts with both male and female patients. Patients across genders tend to prefer women physicians to males, in primary care (Roter et al., 2002; Roter, 1998) and in emergency room settings (Green et al., 2016). Male physicians tend to be more authoritative, more structured, and less responsive to patient cues (Roter & Hall, 2004; Hall et al., 2014). They tend to speak louder and be more "expansive" in their body language (Mast et al. 2008, p. 2016). In general, patients preferred physicians who displayed "gender typical" body language. However, overall, a more typically "female communication style" was preferred by all patients, male and female (Mast et al., 2008). This was particularly true in the emergency room and inpatient setting, whereas there was no difference in satisfaction in the outpatient setting (Hall et al., 2014). Perhaps this is because patients generally have more choice of physician in the outpatient setting, and those choosing male physicians are more in tune with that interaction style.

My mentor, Dr Sidney Feldman, used to say, "There are two people in the room, and you have to care for both of them." In a physician-patient interaction both parties are co-creating the encounter. So how does gender affect the perception of the clinical encounter when doctor and patient are the same or different genders? Women patients are more likely to choose their physicians and will pick female over male practitioners almost twice as often. Interestingly, women patients who specifically chose to have women primary care physicians are the most likely to be disappointed by their physicians' actual behaviour, while male patients who chose female physicians were the most satisfied. There seems to be a high value placed on female physicians' patient centredness by female patients and a concomitant increased risk for disappointment (Roter et al., 2002; Hall et al., 2015). The interaction between patient's gender and physician's gender did not seem to affect the level of patient-centred communication, i.e., the physicians were not more likely to be more or less patient centred in their communication style depending on the sex of their patients (Zandbelt et al., 2006; Schmittdiel et al., 2000). Both male and female physicians respond to women patients' tendency to ask more questions, request more information, receive more counselling and preventive services, and have more participatory visits (Bertakis & Azari, 2012).

Same sex doctor-patient dyads do, however, reinforce the gender typical communication styles. Medical visits between female physicians and female patients were characterized by longer encounter length and more equal patient and physician contributions to the medical dialogue than were visits with all other gender combinations. Medical visits between male physicians and male patients were characterized by the shortest visit time and the highest level of physician verbal dominance (Roter & Hall, 2004).

While both men and women patients prefer a practice style more typical of women, they paradoxically tend to reward male physicians who display a patient-centred style more than they do woman physicians with the same level of patient centeredness (Hall et al., 2014). They feel more positively about a standardized male physician actor in an interaction than with the exact same interaction recorded with a female physician actor (Hall et al., 2015). It is as if patients expect and demand a certain level of patient-centredness from women but are surprised and pleased when men display these characteristics. They attribute patient-centred behaviour to being "a good woman" in women but to being a "good doctor" in men (Hall et al., 2015). Perhaps Dr Kirk is still in some ways correct. Women patients have very high expectations for their women doctors.

Are these skills in communication, attention to the patients' medical and psychosocial information, and better partnering with the patients something inborn? Are male physicians doomed to be poorer at these skills, the way men are predisposed to red-green colour blindness? Or is this a cultural phenomenon and amenable to training? There is the interesting but instructive phenomenon of patient satisfaction and patient-centred communication skills in obstetrics and gynecology. Two separate studies showed that male OB/GYN's were more patient centred than their female colleagues (Hall & Roter, 2002). It seems that in this specialty, where women physicians are strongly preferred for a variety of societal and cultural reasons, the men of the specialty have adjusted to their patients' preferred communication style. I believe that happens in order to compete for patients. Without the option of having male patients in OB, men have had to adjust their style to be more in concordance with what their female patients prefer. These skills are not immutable parts of the psyche; they are culture bound and trainable phenomena.

There is a price to pay for being more patient centred, however. How do women physicians deal with the patient's increased expectation that they will spend more time and psychic energy caring for them than their male counterparts? It is not really known, but one way is probably that they pay for it. Many female family physicians work part time.

While this often reflects their increased demands as family caregivers, even women physicians working over 40 hours/week made less than their male counterparts. Women tend to see fewer patients per hour than their male colleagues but see patients more often (Dollin, 2002).

Roter (1998) suggests that many women choose to limit their practice hours because of the increased emotional demands of their patients:

> Interestingly, female physicians working part-time were found to conduct even longer visits than their female counterparts working on a full-time basis. By assuming part time status, these physicians are in some part relieved of the time pressures of a full patient panel and thereby free to conduct longer visits without the stress of being perpetually behind schedule. (p. 1096)

This practice pattern has certainly been true for me, and I have always seen myself as a low-volume, high-quality practitioner. I cannot bring myself to practise what I consider to be an impoverished form of practice, McMedicine. I want to give my patients the full, gourmet family medicine experience because I have more fun that way. I supplement my office practice income by doing intrapartum obstetrics, not only because I love it but because it is lucrative. And then there is my unfortunate teaching addiction, another way I have chosen to enjoy my practice more but make less money.

One of the rewards of doing good work is getting to do more good work. At one point in my practice I realized that I was getting multiple referrals from private psychotherapists when their patients ran out of insurance or money for therapy. This happened because they knew that while not a therapist, I would at least deal with their clients' psychosocial issues. I also know that when a valued consultant says, "I *need* you to take this patient," it is not going to be a simple case. Taking charge of these often complex patients is the quid pro quo I pay for my quick access to consults and good phone advice. My patients appreciate my commitment and my willingness to go the extra mile for them. Perhaps I really need and value that appreciation and that is how I choose to be "paid."

In my experience as a teacher, it appears that the difference in practice styles between men and women is diminishing over time. *CanMeds Roles* (Frank et al., 2015) are the medical education framework that guides the essential competencies for medical education across all the Royal College specialties. CanMeds and the College of Family Physicians of

Canada's Six Skill Dimensions for Evaluation (College of Family Physicians of Canada, 2009) define competencies that strongly favour a patient-centred approach to care, the traditional strong suit of women doctors. With the introduction of the doctor-patient communication role and collaboration role in CanMeds and patient-centered approach and communication skills skill dimensions in family medicine, both men and women are being trained to be more patient centred. Perhaps more importantly they are being taught, assessed, and evaluated on their patient-centred skills. We know that communication skills and patient-centred care is highly trainable (Brown & Bylund, 2008). This is particularly true in family medicine where they are highly valued. When I started, women were told that they had to be "as tough as the boys" to succeed in medicine. Maybe now the men have to be "as warm and communicative as the girls" to practise in the twenty-first century.

Historically, the healing arts were a woman's domain, and people's illnesses were cared for by women healers, nurses, witches, and traditional midwives. When the rise of scientific medicine started in the seventeenth and eighteenth century, male physicians sought to separate and distinguish themselves from traditional female healers. They did this by valuing the traditional male traits of authoritativeness, logic, and rational discourse. Later, the scientific method and evidence-based medicine became a dominant model in the practice of medicine. But the last 50 years have demonstrated that this stereotypically male approach is not what is best for patients. Indeed:

> medicine, unlike many other male-stereotypic professions, actually requires physicians to possess a combination of stereotypically "masculine" and "feminine" qualities. The masculine qualities include competence, authority, expertise, independence, and self-confidence, while the feminine qualities include warmth, sensitivity, a caring attitude, a relationship orientation, and interpersonal responsiveness. (Hall et al., 2015)

So maybe the times are really changing; maybe the women have taken over. We have hijacked the profession. This is not just because we are growing to be the majority of physicians but in the sense that traditional feminine values are now becoming core to medical education and practice. It is now time for both physicians and patients to leave aside gender stereotypes. It is time for us to accept the balance of talents and skills that all physicians brings to their roles without labelling them "male" or "female." I believe that we are moving in that direction.

REFERENCES

Bertakis, K.D., & Azari, R. (2012, Mar). Patient-centered care: The influence of patient and resident physician gender and gender concordance in primary care. *Journal of Women's Health (2002), 21*(3), 326–33. https://doi.org/10.1089/jwh.2011.2903 Medline:22150099

Brown, R.F., & Bylund, C.L. (2008, Jan). Communication skills training: Describing a new conceptual model. *Academic Medicine: Journal of the Association of American Medical College, 83*(1), 37–44. https://doi.org/10.1097/ACM.0b013e31815c631e Medline:18162748

College of Family Physicians of Canada. (2009). *Defining competence for the purposes of certification by the College of Family Physicians of Canada: The new evaluation objectives in family medicine*. Mississauga, ON: College of Family Physicians of Canada.

Dollin, J. (2002, Jan). The feminization of family medicine: How is the health-care system influenced. *The Canadian Journal of Continuing Medical Education*, 138–45. Retrieved from http://www.stacommunications.com/journals/cme/2002/01-january/cmejan02feminization.pdf

Frank, J.R., Snell, L., & Sherbino, J.E. (2015). *Royal College: Publications. CanMEDS 2015 Physician Competency Framework*. Ottawa: Royal College of Physicians and Surgeons of Canada; Retrieved from http://www.royalcollege.ca/rcsite/canmeds/resources/canmeds-publications-e.

Green, K., Wysocki, J., Espinosa, J., & Scali, V. (2016). The relationship of provider gender to patient satisfaction in the emergency setting: A survey approach and a call for future mixed quantitative-qualitative approaches. *Mathews Journal of Emergency Medicine,1*(1), 001.

Hall, J.A., Gulbrandsen, P., & Dahl, F.A. (2014, Jun). Physician gender, physician patient-centered behavior, and patient satisfaction: A study in three practice settings within a hospital. *Patient Education and Counseling, 95*(3), 313–18. https://doi.org/10.1016/j.pec.2014.03.015 Medline:24731957

Hall, J.A., & Roter, D.L. (2002, Dec). Do patients talk differently to male and female physicians? A meta-analytic review. *Patient Education and Counseling, 48*(3), 217–24. https://doi.org/10.1016/S0738-3991(02)00174-X Medline:12477606

Hall, J.A., Roter, D.L., Blanch-Hartigan, D., Mast, M.S., & Pitegoff, C.A. (2015). How patient-centered do female physicians need to be? Analogue patients' satisfaction with male and female physicians' identical behaviors. *Health communication, 30*(9), 894–900. https://doi.org/10.1080/10410236.2014.900892

Henderson, J.T., & Weisman, C.S. (2001, Dec). Physician gender effects on preventive screening and counseling: An analysis of male and female patients' health care experiences. *Medical Care, 39*(12), 1281–92. https://doi.org/10.1097/00005650-200112000-00004 Medline:11717570

Mast, M.S., Hall, J.A., Köckner, C., & Choi, E. (2008, Dec). Physician gender affects how physician nonverbal behavior is related to patient satisfaction. *Medical Care, 46*(12), 1212–18. https://doi.org/10.1097/MLR.0b013e31817e1877 Medline:19300310

Roter, D. L. (1998). Choices: Biomedical ethics and women's health why physician gender matters in shaping the physician-patient relationship. *Journal of Women's Health, 7*(9), 1093–7.

Roter, D.L., & Hall, J.A. (2004). Physician gender and patient-centered communication: A critical review of empirical research. *Annual Review of Public Health, 25*(1), 497–519. https://doi.org/10.1146/annurev.publhealth.25.101802.123134 Medline:15015932

Roter, D.L., Hall, J.A., & Aoki, Y. (2002, Aug 14). Physician gender effects in medical communication: A meta-analytic review. *JAMA, 288*(6), 756–64. https://doi.org/10.1001/jama.288.6.756 Medline:12169083

Schmittdiel, J., Grumbach, K., Selby, J.V., & Quesenberry, C.P., Jr. (2000, Nov). Effect of physician and patient gender concordance on patient satisfaction and preventive care practices. *Journal of General Internal Medicine, 15*(11), 761–9. https://doi.org/10.1046/j.1525-1497.2000.91156.x Medline:11119167

Zandbelt, L.C., Smets, E.M.A., Oort, F.J., Godfried, M.H., & de Haes, H.C.J.M. (2006, Aug). Determinants of physicians' patient-centred behaviour in the medical specialist encounter. *Social Science & Medicine (1982), 63*(4), 899–910. https://doi.org/10.1016/j.socscimed.2006.01.024 Medline:16530904

SECTION FIVE

Female Doctors in Canada: Futures

The issues explored in this volume reflect a preliminary assessment and the beginning of a conversation of the female doctor's place in the contemporary Canadian health care system. Clearly complex, and obviously critical in some cases, they remind Canadians that the system may in some ways militate against a truly positive outcome for those who shape the system on the ground. Conversely, some of the authors in this volume have made the case for the subtle influence female physicians have had on the culture of medicine, particularly in advocating for the need for improved work-life balance and physician wellness. In this section, we note some ways that policy, structure, and expectations can be better moulded for female to the benefit of all physicians and their patients. Even so, it seems evident that much more study and analysis will be necessary in this important area of health care.

12 Female Doctors in Canada: The Way Forward

EARLE WAUGH, SHELLEY ROSS, AND SHIRLEY SCHIPPER

A Look Back, a Look Ahead

The editors of this volume find much of challenge within these pages, and we are grateful for those who have taken time from busy careers to provide us with their insights. Increasingly, we have become conscious of the flux medicine is in and the strains it puts on both the system and its participants. We have asked family physicians to look over this manuscript and have received very positive responses from them. For most, the material opens vistas not usually conceptualized in this manner, and we are grateful for the suggestions for additional work to be done. We collectively hope that this book encourages a new generation of medical policymakers, planners, and educational specialists to turn their skills to the area – their ideas will help shape better medicine in the decades ahead.

In the course of our work, we have encountered other issues: issues that some regard as pressing and others regard as tangential. In this section of the book, therefore, we have elected to gather these suggestions into three interrelated areas and to challenge colleagues across Canada to engage with them. The three areas can be summarized as policy, culture, and education. In what follows, we summarize dimensions of these areas as best we can, based on our preliminary research and the discussions that have arisen out of shaping this volume.

Policy

The stresses within the system of medicine are thrown in relief as researchers begin to examine what policy revisions have to be made for women to flourish as physicians. Discussions of patchwork changes already applied point out their ineffectiveness; the system still seems to militate against women physicians living fruitful and vibrant lives while pursuing a medical career. One issue that surfaces repeatedly is the nature of the medical system itself: the lock-step model that is in place no longer fits the structural changes brought about by society's demands. This is evident as medical systems move increasingly to a collaborative model, pushed by both women and men in medical careers who want to have a good work-life balance.

Women appear much more accepting of this development, and as health institutions embrace a collaborative model, it would appear that women physicians find it much more amenable to their interests. Our team sees much work to be done in researching, evaluating, and rolling out the widespread adoption of collaborative approaches to health care delivery models. From our discussions, it would appear that women physicians in particular find these approaches accommodate their concerns to a much greater degree than the current model.

Leadership among women physicians, with sufficient numbers of female executives to make the system compatible and attractive, is another topic often encountered. Most studies on roles argue that this area of concern will not change overnight – that they currently are in flux – but they also note that change requires widespread commitment from many levels of society. Changing the system will necessarily include government. We would add that tandem societal change will likely be necessary to effectively reorient the medical system. For example, feminism has had a marked impact on career options for women generally, and the movement has unleashed forces that have clearly outstripped the cultural growth of Canada's medical systems. A genuine evaluation will need to be made of the ways in which the benefits of that movement can be maximized for women in medicine.

On the other hand, the evidence suggests that success as a woman physician may not always be shaped by the system; some writers in this book articulate that their success may not be the norm. Yet research will have to tell us whether one woman's success may not be replicable because of contemporary realities and quick shifts in society. In some scenarios technology will render some kinds of practice obsolete, and researchers will need to determine if the envisioned changes will lead to the desired goal: a more effective system within which women can succeed.

Women physicians report constantly having to compromise their roles as wives, mothers, and custodians of the aged to keep their careers thriving. In this case, policies related to health institutions may well need wholesale review. The point is that health care organizational structures, such as hospitals and school systems, may need to be redesigned to include women physicians with families. For example, in-hospital day-care facilities or nearby primary schools could well support women's goals of caring for patients while caring for their families. This kind of deliberate centralized support model may alleviate some of the stresses faced by female physicians and provide a productive environment for a wholesome career for Canadian women.

Medical Culture and Change

Cultural changes in Canada indicate that norms and values are evolving. The renaissance of Indigenous peoples and the impact of the Truth and Reconciliation Commission on future initiatives is only the most recent and obvious of several. Although medical culture has never been a studied feature of medical training, it is evident that adjustments will need to be made to accommodate the new situation the country is facing. Leadership diversity in medicine needs people with cultural skills to handle the transitions that are coming, and women will fundamentally need to be an energized element in those changes.

This suggests that research is required into issues such as lifestyle so that women's interests and needs can find a place within the system. So, for example, we should no longer ignore family life as a key component in physicians' well-being. There is much incidental evidence of this fact. But with a few exceptions at some more progressive medical schools, work-life balance has no designated place in medical curriculum. In discussions with women physicians this is revealed as a vital problem: for female physicians, and probably also for male, the system *should not* depreciate the importance of a supportive partner in a doctor's successful career. Any strategy for women physicians' well-being needs to take into account the social side directly and cogently. It should not be an add-on attached to handling oneself as a professional.

While it seems true that Canadian women are now having far fewer children, the reasons for this may not be as obvious as they appear. Some evidence suggests that this has been regarded as a lifestyle choice only. But it may not be. It could be a sign that some women do not regard children as the only or principal goal of a successful life. But at the very least, in-depth research needs to be undertaken to determine the shifts that are taking place in this area of social life.

Studies identify ways that culture affects women, but few look at the impact of culture on women of alternative cultures. For example, IMG women carry the legacy of cultural matters with them (think of the hijab or niqab, or of Indigenous differences in family structure); many of these are challenged by Canadian society. Yet it will not do to argue that all women from other cultures must accommodate themselves to living in one culture while they practise and to another when they are at home. A more responsible way would be to find accommodation within a wider system of health care.

Education

In the systems of medicine that appear on the horizon, much greater scope will be given to mentoring. In medical training, discussions have identified strengthening this process by both increasing its role and extending its practice. The mentoring process is usually perceived as a strength of women. As medicine increasingly moves in this direction, women's skills in the process will increase in value. Greater scope is needed at the training level to increase the importance and value of this mentoring process.

Despite a demonstrated capacity to act as good mentors, many women do not have the opportunity because of the lack of women in higher level administrative roles in medical schools and professional organizations. While this trend has been openly acknowledged, there is less emphasis on how to fix it. Studies confirm that the medical system does not stress leadership roles for women. Research is needed, therefore, to determine whether an early emphasis in training should be given to the development of leadership skills among women. Tools for development are available for this purpose, and perhaps educational policy needs to raise them to an open level and apply them at an overt level. Further, education at the continuing professional development level could be multifaceted, targeting both women (encouraging them to pursue leadership roles) and system issues (general educational sessions aimed at revealing underlying assumptions and biases against women in senior leadership positions).

We have long known that medicine has favoured the male person as the norm for medical research; it is a trend reaching back to the Middle Ages. However, discussions indicate that medical education might be more sensitive to women's interests if it used more female examples and deliberately feminized the curriculum around women's prerogatives and women's health. Diversifying the educational models may well have a salutary effect on the broad range of learning that must go on in training a good doctor.

Another aspect of medical culture change that arose in this book was the difference in patient expectations of female versus male physicians. Perle Feldman discusses how 25 years ago, patients consistently expressed a preference for male physicians (perceiving them as more competent), but that trend has shifted. In primary care and emergency room care, research has shown that patients prefer female physicians.

Why the preference? Patients and researchers have found that female physicians spend longer with patients and have a more patient-centred approach. Female physicians are more likely to ask questions than their male counterparts, and they give their patients more opportunities to engage in the clinical encounter through talking and asking questions of their physician. In several studies, this "female communication style" was preferred by both male and female patients.

Surprisingly, this expectation of female physicians can also set these physicians up for criticism. Patients expect more time, engagement, and warmth from their female physicians, and will judge harshly if they feel they have not received adequate levels of these "feminine" elements. However, male physicians are not held to the same standard, and are praised for showing even a minimal amount of patient-centred care.

How will these differences in patient expectations affect the future of medical practice and medical education? In her chapter, Feldman speculates that with the advent of competency-based education and its concurrent increased emphasis on the soft skills of communication and patient-centredness, traditional feminine values are becoming more prevalent in medical education. Her hope is that as good communication and patient-centredness become a fundamental part of medical education, we will no longer talk about these skills as stereotypical gender behaviours, but rather as key components of being a good physician.

Finally, medical education must incorporate, even emphasize, new models of care, rather than reinforcing traditional models that focus on the isolated individual. Research should be undertaken to determine how the appropriation of other solutions, such as group practices, job sharing, part-time possibilities and collaborative care, will impact the system – not just patient outcomes but also job satisfaction among women professionals. In that way, we might get a much more rounded view of the potentials for women in the field.

These represent only a fraction of the issues that surfaced during preparation for this book. We look forward to engaging policymakers, educators and analysts as they wrestle with what will obviously be major changes to Canada's health system.

Contributors

(Please note that there are two authors named Dr. Shelley Ross. Their respective chapters are included after their names below.)

Dr Cheri Bethune is a family physician and medical educator from Memorial University. She is a previous recipient of the Newfoundland and Labrador Medical Association's Primary Healthcare Researcher of the Year. Her recent focus has been on capacity building in research for rural preceptors.

Dr Janet Dollin is a community family physician who is currently an associate professor in the University of Ottawa, Department of Family Medicine. She is the past president of the Federation of Medical Women of Canada. Her women's health initiatives include the Women's Health Fellowship, as well as research and advocacy in HPV prevention. She is currently part of Cancer Care Ontario's cervical screening advisory group.

Dr Deena M. Hamza is a postdoctoral fellow in the Department of Family Medicine at the University of Alberta, in a joint position with the College of Family Physicians of Canada. Her Mitacs-funded postdoctoral fellowship focuses on improving the quality of medical education to ensure the social accountability of future physicians. Dr Hamza's doctoral research focused on models of care in the Department of Psychiatry at the University of Alberta. Much of her research focused on using available resources to provide increased access and support for mental health prevention and early intervention initiatives, particularly for youth. Throughout her graduate work and in her fellowship, Dr Hamza has applied her expertise in mixed methodology and statistics.

Dr Perle Feldman, MDCM, CCFP, FCFP, MHPE, directs the post-graduate program for family medicine at North York General Hospital and is an associate professor at the University of Toronto.

Dr Erin Fredericks is an assistant professor of sociology at St Thomas University in Fredericton, New Brunswick. Her research examines gendered experiences of health and illness.

Dr Kathleen Gartke, FRCSC, is an orthopaedic surgeon at the Ottawa Hospital (with a special interest in the foot and ankle) and an assistant professor at the University of Ottawa. She is a longstanding member of the Federation of Medical Women of Canada executive (a past president) and currently serves as national treasurer. Now in semi-retirement, she is the medical lead at the Ottawa Hospital for patient experience and focuses much of her time on patient safety and continuous quality improvement.

Dr Mamta Gautam is an Ottawa-based psychiatrist, with a special expertise in physician health, physician leadership, and women in medicine. An internationally renowned physician, coach, author, and keynote speaker, she is the recipient of multiple prestigious awards recognizing her pioneering contribution to these areas of medicine. She is also the president and CEO of PEAK MD, a company focused on enhancing leadership resilience and keeping well professionals well.

Dr Gillian Kernaghan is the president and CEO of St. Joseph's Health Care London. She has 23 years of senior health care leadership experience and practised family medicine for 26 years. As a past president of the Canadian Society of Medical Leaders, she has a passion for leadership development.

Monica Olsen is a Toronto-based organization effectiveness consultant, with a special expertise in physician leadership and workplace relationships. A nationally popular seminar leader, coach, and author, she is also the president of Olsen and Associates Consulting, a company focused on cultivating leadership development at all levels.

Dr Shelley Ross (Chapter 8) graduated from the University of Alberta Faculty of Medicine in 1974. She went on to receive a certification and fellowship in family medicine and spent her entire career as a full service family physician in Burnaby, BC, where she had a special interest in obstetrics and women's health. She developed her interest in medical politics through the Federation of Medical Women of Canada, the Medical Women's International Association, the Doctors of BC, and the Canadian Medical Association.

Dr Shelley Ross (co-editor; author of Chapters 1, 4, 12) is an associate professor and medical education researcher in the Department of Family Medicine at the University of Alberta. She obtained her doctorate from the Department of Educational Psychology and Leadership Studies at the University of Victoria, where she studied the effects of varying levels of motivation on academic achievement. Dr Ross has been recognized for her work in improving health professional education practices by the University of Alberta (Information Technology Excellence Award, 2015; David Cook Award for Education Innovation, 2012), the Alberta College of Family Physicians (Recognition of Excellence Award, 2011), and the Royal College of Physicians and Surgeons of Canada (Royal College Accredited CPD Provider Innovation Award, 2015; International Conference on Residency Education Top Paper, 2013).

Dr Inge Schabort, MB ChB, CCFP, FCFP, is an associate professor of family medicine and the international medical graduate (IMG) coordinator and academic half day coordinator at McMaster University. She practises as a full-time family physician at the Stonechurch clinical teaching unit at McMaster, and she tutors evidence-based medicine, quality assurance, and behavioural sciences in the residency program. She teaches in and developed curriculum for the provincial pre-residency IMG program in Ontario.

Dr Shirley Schipper is an associate professor with the Department of Family Medicine at the University of Alberta. Dr Schipper was previously the academic and medical director for the Grey Nuns Family Medicine Academic Teaching Clinic, where she also has a clinical practice. She is currently the vice dean of education for the Faculty of Medicine and Dentistry at the University of Alberta. At the national level, she is a member of the chairs for accreditation group and a member of the accreditation committee for the College of Family Physicians of Canada.

Dr Heather Stanley is a historian of the body, sexuality, medicine, and gender. Her most current work examines the history of the married sexual body during Canada's baby boom. She has also published work on medical professionalization and gender in Canada and Britain. She is an assistant professor at Vancouver Island University.

Dr Setorme Tsikata is an assistant clinical professor with the Department of Family Medicine at the University of Alberta in Edmonton. She is an assessor for the provincial physician assessment program, which licenses international medical graduates (IMGs) for independent practice through the College of Physicians and Surgeons of Alberta. She is also a member of the Patient Education Committee of the College of Family Physicians of Canada. She is the current Region II representative for the Federation of Medical Women of Canada, which has opened diverse opportunities for mentoring medical students, residents, and IMGs. In addition to her family medicine certification from Dalhousie University, she has a fellowship in women's health from the University of Ottawa, a MSc in health services research from the Netherlands Institute of Health Sciences, Erasmus University, Rotterdam, and a MBChB from Kwame Nkrumah University of Science and Technology, Ghana. She belongs to a group family practice in Spruce Grove, Alberta, and often presents lectures in her areas of interests (including palliative care, women's health, patient-centred medicine, culturally appropriate medicine, refugee health), internationally, particularly in Ghana where she is originally from. She lives with her husband and two children in Edmonton.

Dr Earle H. Waugh is a professor emeritus of religious studies and of the Centre for Health and Culture in the Department of Family Medicine at the University of Alberta. In recent years, he has concentrated on cultural competency in medicine, with, for example, *Culturally Competent Skills for Health Care Professionals: A Workbook* (Brush Education, 2014). He lectures and consults widely on health care and culture and has provided seminars for hospitals, pharmacy seniors, graduate physicians, and health care professionals throughout Alberta. His longtime commitment to education about minority groups was recognized in 2005 with the prestigious Salvos Prelorentzos Award for Peace Education by Project Ploughshares and the 2010 Friend of Pharmacy of the Year award by the Alberta College of Pharmacist.